Praise for...

Miller's Review of Critical Vaccine Studies, Volume 2

"Neil Miller's new book, *Miller's Review of Critical Vaccine Studies, Volume 2,* is a tremendous addition to the incredible material that appeared and was reviewed in the first volume. What he demonstrates clearly from these reviews is that we have to get past the Madison Avenue hype of the pharmaceutical makers and beyond the empty praises of 'safety and effectiveness' that are being promoted, and other falsehoods about these injections. As I tell people constantly, you can get vaccinated but cannot get unvaccinated. We are now seeing side effects that we never even conceived of in the beginning, and many are long-term effects that severely impact children and adults regarding acute, subacute, and especially chronic diseases. Often, doctors either do not know about these vaccine side effects or deny them to protect themselves. These two books, Volumes I and II, should open the eyes of critical thinkers. With the COVID-19 injections we are now in a different ballgame, which he describes so well. It is terrifying that these mRNA injections have been included in the new vaccine schedule. Neil's book also discusses the attempt to use vaccines as birth control (or population control) devices. One topic he covers well is what most people, even doctors, fail to mention, which is vaccine contamination. Everyone, not just parents, should read and study these books by Neil Miller before even considering having vaccines."
—*Russell L. Blaylock, MD, Neurosurgeon (retired)*

"As a holistic pediatrician I regularly discuss many aspects of vaccines with parents and parents-to-be. Consumers have a right to detailed scientific information before consenting to vaccination, a set of procedures that should always be presented as elective, not mandatory, and that should be accompanied by full informed consent. The medical profession and our government agencies are falling short when it comes to providing accurate, accessible information to assist people in their decision-making regarding vaccines. Doing one's due diligence is much easier since we have Neil Z. Miller's books to turn to. Since they were published, I have had his *Vaccine Safety Manual* and *Miller's Review of Critical Vaccine Studies: 400 Important Scientific Papers Summarized...*on the short list of resources I provide to parents who need access to dependable, user-friendly information. And now we have summaries of 400 more studies! It's obvious that Mr. Miller has dedicated many hours to researching and writing this book. He has included more information on some topics covered previously, including influenza and measles/ MMR, and also reviews more recent science on Covid vaccines and related subjects, as well as delving into other fascinating areas such as how the intestinal microbiome interacts with vaccine effectiveness. This book is another invaluable tool for those seeking to learn the truth about vaccines. I'm happy to be able to add it to my list of trustworthy references."
—*Janet Levatin, MD, Holistic Pediatrician, Homeopathic Master Clinician; Former clinical instructor in Pediatrics, Harvard Medical School*

"Neil Miller has done it again! His earlier review of 400 scientific research articles was a priceless gift to all researchers studying the adverse effects of vaccines. Here is Volume 2, summarizing 400 more articles, including 96 on the COVID vaccines alone. For those investigators who want to begin with knowing what's out there, this is another must-read that covers the whole territory."
—*Richard Moskowitz, MD*

"In this magnum opus — *Miller's Review of Critical Vaccine Studies, Volume 2* — Neil Miller has painstakingly assembled 400 scientific studies demonstrating that vaccines, including covid vaccines, either lack efficacy or cause harm, or both. Each study has been condensed to one page or less making for quick, easy reading. Most useful is a chapter of 13 studies showing that persons with low levels of vitamin D are at greater risk of contracting covid, being hospitalized and dying than those with high levels of vitamin D. My wish is that this important information be read by the many vaccine proponents who are unaware of this mountain of scientific evidence that questions the notion that vaccines are beyond reproach and entirely safe. For those of us who are vaccine skeptics, with this book we are now well-armed. Let a robust debate begin."
—*Karl Robinson, MD*

"In recent times, we've observed mainstream media predominantly endorsing the vaccination narrative while often stigmatizing those who raise questions. In light of this, the presence of research journalists like Neil Miller becomes invaluable. Through diligent fact-gathering, Miller provides parents and healthcare providers with the necessary information to make informed decisions regarding vaccinations. His latest publication, *Miller's Review of Critical Vaccine Studies, Volume 2,* stands as a monumental achievement deserving widespread recognition and attention."
—*Harry van der Zee, MD*

"Vaccine blindness—the inability to see the less desirable side of vaccines—is a special form of science blindness and certainly predates the tyranny of covid-19. I think it was probably brought to the fore by the 1986 act giving immunity to vaccine manufacturers and the serious collateral damage caused by their products. Where can you turn for the truth, how can you begin to solve a problem like vaccine blindness? The peer-reviewed published research is available, but it is not readily accessible to working scientists and doctors, even less so to the layperson. Who are you going to contact to find the truth? Step forward *Miller's Review of Critical Vaccine Studies, Volume 2.* Neil Miller is one of the truth-tellers amongst us and he has once again brought together the very best vaccine research. He does science a great service in publishing this new volume of the best truth we have. Read, digest and come to your own decisions on the safety of vaccines. Neil Miller gives you this choice."
—*Christopher Exley, PhD, FRSB (Fellowship of the Royal Society of Biology)*

"If you search for vaccine risks or side effects on your favorite search engine, you would be hard-pressed to find information which suggests that the risks may outweigh the benefits for any vaccine—but you will easily find info that either normalizes or minimizes a vaccine's risks. Even all the data on our website, which has been around for almost a decade, is hard to find unless you have our exact web address. *Miller's Review of Critical Vaccine Studies, Volume 2,* just like the first volume, is the perfect solution to the conundrum of the 'vaccine risks void' and offers more than enough studies for you to research—right at your fingertips.
—*Shira Miller, MD, Founder and President, Physicians for Informed Consent*

"Patients have the legal right to hear both sides of the debate on vaccine safety and effectiveness but the CDC and most doctors only give the CDC's side of it. Here, Neil Miller gives the other side of the debate that all patients should read before consenting to get any more vaccinations."
—*Richard B. Fox, MD, JD, Physician & Attorney*

"Miller's boundless efforts have again uncovered even more critical vaccine studies that are mostly glossed over or ignored by the medical profession. His post-mortem on the covid 'vaccines' is especially enlightening."
—*John W. Travis, MD, MPH. Author, Wellness Workbook—How to Achieve Enduring Health and Vitality*

Miller's Review of Critical Vaccine Studies, Volume 2

400 More Scientific Papers Summarized for Parents and Researchers

Neil Z. Miller

New Atlantean Press
Santa Fe, New Mexico

Miller's Review of Critical Vaccine Studies, Volume 2

400 More Scientific Papers Summarized for Parents and Researchers

by Neil Z. Miller

ISBN: 978-188121744-2

Cataloging-in-Publication Data

Miller, Neil Z., author.
  Miller's review of critical vaccine studies, volume 2 : 400 more scientific
papers summarized for parents and researchers / Neil Z. Miller.
      p. ; cm.
  Review of critical vaccine studies
  Includes bibliographical references and index.
  ISBN 978-1-881217-44-2
  I. Title. II. Title: Review of critical vaccine studies.
  [DNLM: 1. Vaccination. 2. Vaccines. 3. Biomedical Research. 4. Child.
5. Safety. QW 805]
  RA638
  614.4'7--dc23

            Library of Congress Control Number: 2024942881

Cover photo: Bigstock

Printed in the United States of America

Published by:
New Atlantean Press
PO Box 9638
Santa Fe, NM 87504
www.vacbook.com

*This publication is dedicated
to parents and their children.*

Contents

Foreword

Paul Thomas, MD

I was a board certified pediatrician for 30 years. I graduated from Dartmouth Medical School in 1985 and finished my residency in 1987. I moved to Portland, Oregon the following year. In 1993, I joined Westside Pediatrics, a private group practice in Portland where I worked alongside four other pediatricians.

I am the proud father of ten children, all of whom are fully vaccinated. I was still unaware of vaccine risks when my youngest was born in 1996. I just hadn't woken up yet. I was trained very well that vaccines are "safe and effective." It's what I was taught during my years in medical school, and I believed it. When you're training in pediatrics, you don't get a lot of information on vaccines other than the diseases for which you vaccinate and how horrible they are, and how wonderful it is that we have a vaccine. That's pretty much the extent of it.

When you get into residency, you definitely don't have the time to research things in depth on your own. What you're learning at that point is what to do. You learn protocols, and so with vaccinations I learned what the Academy of Pediatrics (AAP) and the Centers for Disease Control and Prevention (CDC) wanted me to learn.

In 1998, I read Andrew Wakefield's paper which, although not specifically about a link between vaccines and autism, caused me and others to question that very connection. It was my first little wake-up call. I then took a deep dive into studies that presented a different look at the safety and effectiveness of vaccines. It was far different than what I had been taught in school. I began questioning everything I had ever learned about vaccines. More than that, as a pediatrician I had to be willing to acknowledge the possibility that something I was doing to children with the intent of helping them was instead causing them harm.

The first case of regressive autism that I saw as a pediatrician was in 2004. The next year, I saw a second case. Then yet another the following year. The fourth case came in November 2007. I remember it like it was yesterday. I had an appointment to see a two-year-old. He was supposed to be a well kid but he was shaking his head back and forth and the lights were missing from his eyes. It seemed as if nobody was home.

I could no longer do business as usual adhering to the CDC's vaccine schedule for my patients once I became clearly aware of their potential for injury. I approached my partners at Westside Pediatrics and expressed my concerns. They felt it was unethical to de anything other than what they were told by the AAP and CDC. I felt it was unethical to continue the "standard of care" practice of treating vaccination as a one-size-fits-all solution to infectious disease. In 2008, after fifteen years with the group practice, I left and opened my own clinic, Integrative Pediatrics, in Beaverton, Oregon. It was a move necessitated by my continued awakening to the possibility that I was contributing to iatrogenic impairment, no matter how well-intended I may have been.

My new clinic attracted parents of children who had already developed chronic health conditions or developmental disorders. I also began noticing a marked difference in the health of patients whose parents were choosing not to follow the CDC's recommendations. We started seeing that our less vaccinated or unvaccinated children seemed to be healthier than the ones that received all of the shots. I mean, it was palpable; you could just tell.

People often misquote me. They allege that I'm saying, "Vaccines cause autism," but that's not what I'm saying. I'm declaring that I observed vaccinated children regressing into autism at a much higher rate than the unvaccinated. And it wasn't just autism. I was seeing a marked reduction of nearly every type of chronic disease in my unvaccinated kids. I wanted to share this information, so in August 2016 I coauthored a book with Dr. Jennifer Margulis: *The Vaccine-Friendly Plan.* I wanted to empower parents to make their own informed decisions when it came to their children's health. Although I was definitely on the Oregon Medical Board's radar prior to this, publication of my book solidified their resolve to discipline me. My crime? Fully informing the parents of my young patients about the good, the bad, and the ugly regarding vaccines and allowing *them* to decide how they wanted to have vaccines administered, if at all.

The first accusation from the Medical Board came on December 26, 2018. The Board sent me a letter stating that I had provided care related to vaccinations during pregnancy and early childhood that was "not consistent with the CDC, American Academy of Pediatrics, and other evidence-based medicine practices." Looking at my records, I was able to conclude that it was an unsubstantiated allegation. The charge came from someone who wasn't even one of my patients!

In 2019, I worked on a study with Dr. James Lyons-Weiler (and two additional authors) titled "Acute exposure and chronic retention of aluminum in three vaccine schedules and effects of genetic and environmental variation." We compared the acute exposure to aluminum that children receive from the CDC's schedule with that from my "vaccine-friendly plan," which aims to reduce exposure by choosing versions that have a lower dose of aluminum, if available, and otherwise spacing vaccines out so that only one aluminum-containing vaccine is given at a time. It was published in March of 2020.

In November of 2020, Lyons-Weiler and I published another peer-reviewed study using 10 years' worth of data from my practice. We compared the incidence of diagnoses on a wide range of health problems and found that the completely unvaccinated children in my practice were diagnosed at much lower rates than the vaccinated children. Five days following the publication of our study, the Oregon Medical Board suspended my license to practice. A month after that, the journal informed us that an anonymous reader had expressed some concerns about the study. This single reader's comments ultimately led to the journal's decision to retract our paper, leaving Lyons-Weiler and myself bewildered.

On June 3, 2021, I entered into an Interim Stipulated Order with the Board in which I agreed to voluntarily limit my practice to acute care; refrain from engaging in consultations or directing clinic staff with respect to vaccination protocol questions, issues or recommendations; and refrain from performing any research involving patient care pending the completion of the Board's investigation. In 2022, after the Board continued to threaten imposing sanctions, I made the difficult decision to surrender my Oregon license. However, I continue my crusade of vaccine safety awareness by combing through the studies and literature on the subject to share my findings.

I can tell you that most pediatricians are not even aware of the published science that addresses vaccine side effects and injuries. The connection between vaccines and neurodevelopmental, allergic and immune challenges is also not understood by pediatricians, public health officials and parents. The media and professional academies, including governmental and private organizations that are thought to be there to protect our health (AAP, AMA, CDC, NIH, FDA, etc.), are all silent on the most important research done. Professional journals seem to aggressively oppose publishing articles that show problems with vaccines. Many of those that do get published end up being retracted for bogus reasons or no reasons at all.

Enter *Miller's Review of Critical Vaccine Studies*. Volume I covered 400 important scientific papers and summarized them for parents and professionals. Finally, there was one place we could all go to get the actual references and the summaries of the findings. Thousands of hours of research done for us.

Now, Neil Miller has done it again. You are holding the most up-to-date publication, *Miller's Review of Critical Vaccine Studies, Volume II,* summarizing the world literature we need to know about before we choose to vaccinate. This book summarizes 400 additional peer-reviewed scientific papers. It contains the most recent data on vaccinated vs. unvaccinated children and child mortality, covid-19 and cardiovascular events, super-spreaders, measles, and lots more! Indeed, this is a perfect complement to my just released book, *VAX Facts: What to Consider Before Vaccinating.* These books belong on the night stand or coffee table of every critical thinking parent or child caregiver. It is time we have these important conversations about vaccines. Without our proper attention to what is really happening with vaccines, this and future generations of children will suffer greatly.

Introduction

There are literally thousands of studies published in peer-reviewed medical journals that document problems with vaccines. These include studies that confirm poor efficacy or even negative efficacy (when vaccinated people are more likely than the unvaccinated to contract the disease). Other studies provide evidence that vaccines cause serious adverse events, such as an increased risk of developing a neurological disorder or immunological injury.

When I wrote the first book in this series, *Miller's Review of Critical Vaccine Studies* (Volume 1), I summarized 400 important scientific papers that I thought were important for parents and researchers to know about. Some of the topics that I discussed were on mercury, aluminum, allergies, seizures, diabetes, premature infants, cancer and natural infections, conflicts of interest, false studies, and industry control. This book, *Miller's Review of Critical Vaccine Studies*, *Volume 2*, picks up where the last one left off. It continues the trend of summarizing studies that vaccine policymakers, regulators, and even your family doctor are unlikely to share with you. The mainstream media is even less likely to write about these papers. Some of the topics covered in this book include: vaccinated versus unvaccinated children, child mortality, the covid-19 vaccine and cardiovascular events, face masks, obesity, the pertussis vaccine and all-cause mortality, rotavirus, birth control vaccines, and contaminated vaccines.

The studies in this book do not support vaccine safety and effectiveness. Instead, they provide scientific evidence of risks and detriments, confirming adverse side effects or tradeoffs associated with vaccination. For example, the vaccine might decrease the likelihood of contracting a contagious ailment while increasing the odds of developing Guillain-Barré syndrome (paralysis), myocarditis (a serious heart ailment), or death. Other possibilities are narcolepsy, arthritis, depression, or menstrual irregularities. Vaccinated children may also be trading a reduced risk of infections for an increased risk of developmental disorders and chronic diseases that significantly reduce their quality of life.

Most of the studies in this book are peer-reviewed and published in medical journals indexed by the U.S. National Library of Medicine (the world's largest medical library). Many of the studies summarized in this book were published in prestigious or high-impact journals such as the *Journal of the American Medical Association, British Medical Journal, New England Journal of Medicine, Journal of Pediatrics, Journal of Internal Medicine, Journal of Cardiovascular Medicine, Journal of Virology, American Journal of Epidemiology, American Journal of Infection Control, Proceedings of the National Academy of Sciences, International*

Journal of Obesity, Emerging Infectious Diseases, Cancer Causes & Control, Toxicology Reports, JAMA Pediatrics, Lancet, Nature Medicine, Science, European J of Epidemiology, Scientific Reports, Eurosurveillance, Obstetrics & Gynecology, and *Nature.* Of course, this does not mean that studies published in highly-cited journals are more valuable than those published in lesser known journals. All studies must be scrutinized for potential strengths and weaknesses.

The scientific papers in this book are organized into 26 chapters. Each chapter contains several studies on a particular topic, such as covid vaccine effectiveness and treatment, DTP and all-cause mortality, the microbiome, and super-spreaders. Usually, there is one study per page although some pages contain two or three studies. At the top of each page is a headline. Next, there is a direct quote taken from the study. This is followed by the scientific citation. Finally, I use bullet points to summarize, in my own words, pertinent findings in the paper.

Important findings from each scientific paper reviewed in this book are provided for quick reference and to counterbalance the many well-publicized studies touting the advantages of vaccination. I endeavored to remain free from bias at all times, with one caveat — my goal was to summarize studies that shed light on poorly publicized and unpopular aspects of vaccination. For readers with a scientific background, I included odds ratios, relative incidence and other statistical measures when p-values achieved significance. Confidence intervals can be found in the original studies.

The findings in some of the summarized studies may conflict with those in other studies. There are many reasons why studies on the same topic might have contrary results. Studies may be poorly designed or conducted by researchers with conflicts of interest that bias their findings.

I highly recommend reading the actual complete studies, which often contain supplementary figures, tables, data and discussions not included in my summaries. Some scientific papers are freely available from the medical journals that published them. Others are fee-based although an abstract of the paper is almost always available at no cost.

Studies that support vaccination are not included in this book. You can find supportive information by visiting official websites of the Centers for Disease Control and Prevention (CDC), the Food and Drug Administration (FDA), the World Health Organization (WHO), vaccine manufacturers, and by conducting your own search in medical journals. I encourage you to do your own careful research to better understand the benefits and risks of vaccination.

Neil Z. Miller
Medical Research Journalist

Vaccinated vs. Unvaccinated and Child Mortality

The first four studies in this chapter compared vaccinated and unvaccinated children. The first study was based on more than 2,000 electronic medical records obtained from three medical practices in the United States. Vaccinated children were two to four times more likely than unvaccinated children to have been diagnosed with developmental delays, asthma, ear infections, and gastrointestinal disorders.

The second study had a sample population of more than 1,500 people. Vaccinated children were four to 27 times more likely than unvaccinated children to have been diagnosed with allergies, autism, gastrointestinal disorders, asthma, ADHD, and ear infections. In addition, unvaccinated breastfed children had the best health outcomes while vaccinated non-breastfed children had the worst.

The third study found that vaccinated children were significantly more likely than unvaccinated children to have been diagnosed with an ear infection, pneumonia, allergies, ADHD, a learning disability, autism, any chronic illness, and any neuro-developmental disorder. The fourth study found that vaccinated preterm infants were 14 times more likely than unvaccinated children born at term to have been diagnosed with a neurodevelopmental disorder.

The last four studies in this chapter looked at the relationship between vaccines and pediatric mortality rates. The fifth study did a linear regression of the most highly developed nations and found that those that require more vaccines for their infants tend to have higher infant mortality rates. This study corroborated an earlier study by the same authors. The sixth study found that developed nations that require that most neonatal vaccines (hepatitis B and tuberculosis) have the worst neonatal, infant, and under age five mortality rates.

The seventh study analyzed 2605 infant deaths reported to the Vaccine Adverse Event Reporting System (VAERS) and found that 58% clustered within three days post-vaccination and 78% within seven days post-vaccination, confirming that infant deaths tend to occur in temporal proximity to vaccine administration, a statistically significant finding ($p < 0.00001$).

The final study in this chapter analyzed data on millions of infants and found that twice as many died after receiving a pentavalent vaccine (designed to protect against five diseases: diphtheria, tetanus, pertussis, hepatitis B, and Hib) compared to infants vaccinated with DTP.

1.

Vaccinated children are significantly more likely than unvaccinated children to be diagnosed with developmental delays and other adverse health conditions

"In this study, based on a convenience sample of children born into one of three distinct pediatric medical practices, higher odds ratios were observed within the vaccinated versus unvaccinated group for developmental delays, asthma and ear infections."

Hooker BS, Miller NZ. **Analysis of health outcomes in vaccinated and unvaccinated children: developmental delays, asthma, ear infections and gastrointestinal disorders.** *SAGE Open Med* 2020 May 27; 8: 2050312120925344.

- In this study, vaccinated children were compared to unvaccinated children during the first year of life for later incidence of developmental delays, asthma, ear infections and gastrointestinal disorders.

- Patient data, including vaccination records and diagnoses, were obtained from the electronic medical records of three medical practices in the United States. The sample population consisted of 2,047 children.

- Vaccination before 1 year of age was associated with increased odds of developmental delays (odds ratio, OR = 2.18), asthma (OR = 4.49) and ear infections (OR = 2.13). In secondary analyses, statistical significance was also seen for gastrointestinal disorders.

- In a quartile analysis, higher ORs were observed in Quartiles 3 and 4 (where more vaccine doses were received) for all four health conditions considered, as compared to Quartile 1, which is suggestive of a dose-response relationship.

- Higher ORs were observed for all four health conditions when time permitted for a diagnosis was extended from 3 years of age to 5 years of age.

2.

Vaccinated children are significantly more likely than unvaccinated children to be diagnosed with allergies, asthma, autism, ADHD and other adverse health conditions

"In the study presented here, several acute and chronic adverse health outcomes were found to be more likely in fully and partially vaccinated children as compared to an unvaccinated child population."

Hooker BS, Miller NZ. **Health effects in vaccinated versus unvaccinated children, with covariates for breastfeeding status and type of birth.** *J Transl Sci* 2021 Jun 12; 7: 1-11.

- In this study, vaccinated children were compared to unvaccinated children for the incidence of severe allergies, autism, gastrointestinal disorders, asthma, attention deficit hyperactivity disorder (ADHD), and chronic ear infections.

- Patient data were obtained from a survey given primarily to participants in three US pediatric practices. The sample population was 1,565 children. In a separate analysis, diagnoses were confirmed from electronic medical records.

- Vaccinated children were significantly more likely than unvaccinated children to be diagnosed with severe allergies (odds ratio, OR = 4.31), autism (OR = 5.03), gastrointestinal disorders (OR = 13.8), asthma (OR = 17.6), ADHD (OR = 20.8), and chronic ear infections (OR = 27.8).

- Although partially and fully vaccinated children were significantly more likely than unvaccinated children to have adverse health diagnoses, odds ratios were considerable more elevated in the fully vaccinated cohort, suggestive of a dose-response relationship or synergisitic toxicity.

- Unvaccinated breastfed children had the best health outcomes while vaccinated non-breastfed children had the worst (Table 9). Unvaccinated children delivered vaginally had the best health outcomes while vaccinated children delivered via cesarean section had the worst (Table 10).

- Vaccinated children were less likely to be diagnosed with chickenpox.

3.

Vaccinated children are significantly more likely than unvaccinated children to develop attention deficit hyperactivity disorder, learning disabilities, and autism

"In conclusion, vaccinated homeschool children were found to have a higher rate of allergies and neurodevelopmental disorders than unvaccinated homeschool children."

Mawson AR, Ray BD, et al. **Pilot comparative study on the health of vaccinated and unvaccinated 6- to 12-year-old U.S. children.** *J Transl Sci* 2017 April 24; 3(3): 1-12.

- In this study, 666 mothers of children educated at home completed an anonymous online questionnaire pertaining to their 6- to 12-year-old children regarding pregnancy-related factors, birth history, vaccinations received, physician-diagnosed illnesses, medications used, and health services.

- This study was designed to 1) compare vaccinated and unvaccinated children on several health outcomes, and 2) determine whether there's a statistically significant link between vaccines and neurodevelopmental disorders after making adjustments for other factors.

- Vaccinated children were significantly less likely than the unvaccinated to have had chickenpox (odds ratio, OR = 0.26) and pertussis (OR = 0.30) but significantly more likely to have been diagnosed with otitis media, a painful ear infection (OR = 3.8) and pneumonia (OR = 5.9).

- Vaccinated children were significantly more likely than the unvaccinated to have been diagnosed with allergies (OR = 3.9), ADHD (OR = 4.2), a learning disability (OR = 5.2), autism (OR = 4.2), any neurodevelopmental disorder (OR = 3.7), and any chronic illness (OR = 2.4).

- Boys were significantly more likely than girls to have been diagnosed with autism (OR = 4.3) and any neurodevelopmental disorder (OR = 2.3). In an adjusted analysis, neurodevelopmental disorders were much more likely in vaccinated preterm babies (OR = 6.6) and non-white children (OR = 2.4).

4.

Vaccinated preterm infants have a high risk of neurodevelopmental disorders; preterm birth without vaccination is not linked to neurodevelopmental disorders

"Vaccination was found to be significantly and independently associated with neurodevelopmental disorders, whereas preterm birth without vaccination was not. However, vaccination coupled with preterm birth greatly increased the odds of neurodevelopmental disorders over that of vaccination alone, especially compared to being born at term and unvaccinated."

Mawson AR, Bhuiyan A, et al. **Preterm birth, vaccination and neuro-developmental disorders: a cross-sectional study of 6- to 12-year-old vaccinated and unvaccinated children.** *J Transl Sci* 2017 April 24; 3(3): 1-8.

- Preterm birth is associated with neurodevelopmental disorders, including autism. Up to 27% of extremely preterm infants develop symptoms of autism.

- Preterm infants are excluded from pre-licensure studies of pediatric vaccines although after these vaccines are licensed they are given to all infants regardless of gestational age. Thus, the possible role of vaccination in neurodevelopmental disorders among premature infants is unknown.

- This study compared vaccinated and unvaccinated children 6 to 12 years of age who were born prematurely to determine whether there's an association between preterm birth, vaccination, and neurodevelopmental disorders (NDD).

- In unvaccinated children, there was no association between preterm birth and NDD. However, in vaccinated children there was a significant link between NDD and children born at term (odds ratio, OR = 2.7).

- Vaccinated children born preterm were 5 times more likely than vaccinated children born at term to have been diagnosed with NDD (OR = 5.4) and 14 times more likely than unvaccinated children born at term to have been diagnosed with NDD (OR = 14.5).

5.

There is a positive correlation between infant vaccines and infant mortality rates

"There is a positive correlation between infant vaccines and infant mortality rates. This relationship is most pronounced in analyses of the most highly developed homogenous nations but is attenuated in background noise in analyses of nations with heterogeneous socioeconomic variables."

Goldman GS, Miller NZ. **Reaffirming a positive correlation between number of vaccine doses and infant mortality rates: a response to critics.** *Cureus* 2023 Feb 2; 15(2): e34566.

- The authors' previous study found a high correlation ($r = 0.70, p < .0001$) among 30 developed nations: those requiring the most pediatric vaccines tended to have the worst infant mortality rates. Critics of the earlier study claimed that the "full dataset" of all 185 nations should have been analyzed.

- This current paper examined claims made by these critics, and three new investigations were conducted corroborating the authors' original finding.

- The critics' reanalysis of 185 nations was flawed because their dataset mixed developed and Third World nations that have varying rates of vaccination and socioeconomic disparities. In contrast, nations in the Miller-Goldman dataset had high vaccination rates and homogeneity of socioeconomic factors.

- Despite multiple confounders, the critics affirmed a small, positive correlation between infant vaccines and infant mortality rates ($r = 0.16, p < .03$).

- Goldman and Miller provided an odds ratio analysis that controlled for several variables, including child poverty, low birth weight, and breast feeding; none lowered the correlation below 0.62, robustly confirming their original finding.

- Goldman and Miller conducted a sensitivity analysis revealing that when less developed nations are added to the dataset, confounders are introduced.

- A replication study using 2019 data corroborated ($r = 0.45, p = .002$) the positive trend reported in the original 2011 Miller-Goldman study.

6.

There is a positive correlation between childhood vaccines and childhood mortality rates

"There are statistically significant positive correlations between neonatal, infant, and under age five mortality rates of developed nations and the number of early childhood vaccine doses that are routinely given."

Miller NZ, Goldman GS. **Neonatal, infant, and under age five vaccine doses routinely given in developed nations and their association with mortality rates.** *Cureus* 2023 Jul 20; 15(7): e42194.

- In this study, researchers explored potential associations between the number of early childhood vaccine doses required by nations and their neonatal, infant, and under age five mortality rates.

- Developed nations requiring the most childhood vaccines doses tend to have the worst childhood mortality rates.

- Linear regression of neonatal vaccine doses required by developed nations in 2021 yielded statistically significant positive correlations to rates of neonatal mortality ($r = 0.34, p = .017$), infant mortality ($r = 0.46, p = .0008$), and under age five mortality ($r = 0.48, p = .0004$). Results were similar in 2019.

- Linear regression of infant vaccine doses required by developed nations in 2021 yielded statistically significant positive correlations to rates of infant mortality ($r = 0.47, p = .0005$) and under age five mortality ($r = 0.46, p = .0007$). Results were similar in 2019.

- When nations require two versus zero neonatal vaccine doses (hepatitis B and BCG), or many versus fewer infant vaccine doses, there may be unintended consequences that increase childhood mortality.

- Some deaths associated with neonatal vaccines may be delayed, possibly through a priming mechanism or cumulative toxicity that increases the risk of a severe or fatal reaction to subsequently administered vaccines.

7.

Sudden infant deaths reported to VAERS tend to cluster within one week after vaccination

"This study found that a substantial proportion of infant deaths and SIDS cases occurred in temporal proximity to vaccine administration. The excess of deaths during these early post-vaccination periods was statistically significant."

Miller NZ. **Vaccines and sudden infant death: an analysis of the VAERS database 1990-2019 and review of the medical literature.** *Tox Rep* 2021 Jun 24; 8: 1324-35.

- In this paper, the Vaccine Adverse Event Reporting System (VAERS) database was analyzed for an association between infant vaccines and sudden infant deaths. If no relationship exists, SIDS cases should be evenly distributed each day rather than clustering in the early post-vaccination period.

- Of 2605 infant deaths reported to VAERS from 1990-2019, 58% clustered within 3 days post-vaccination and 78% within 7 days post-vaccination, confirming that infant deaths tend to occur in temporal proximity to vaccine administration, a statistically significant finding (p < 0.00001).

- A smaller proportion of total infant deaths were reported on the day of vaccination than on the day after vaccination, suggestive of an incubation period (the time after vaccination to develop the full reaction causing death), evidence that reporting bias cannot fully explain the clustering of deaths.

- Health authorities eliminated "prophylactic vaccination" as an official cause of death, so medical examiners are compelled to misclassify and conceal vaccine-related fatalities under alternate cause-of-death classifications.

- Several theories regarding the pathogenic mechanism behind SIDS cases post-vaccination have been proposed, including the role of inflammatory cytokines as neuromodulators in the infant medulla.

- A review of the medical literature substantiates a link between vaccines and sudden unexplained infant deaths.

8.

The pentavalent vaccine doubles the risk of sudden infant death

"This study demonstrated an increase in reports of sudden unexplained deaths within 72 hours of administering pentavalent vaccine compared to DTP vaccine."

Puliyel J, Kaur J, et al. **Deaths reported after pentavalent vaccine compared with death reported after diphtheria-tetanus-pertussis vaccine: an exploratory analysis.** *Med J DY Patil Vidyapeeth* 2018; 11(2): 99-105.

- In India, there have been newspaper reports of sudden infant deaths shortly after the administration of a newly introduced pentavalent vaccine (designed to protect against 5 diseases: diphtheria, tetanus, pertussis, *Haemophilus influenzae* type B, and hepatitis B).

- In this study, researchers analyzed government data on 25 million infants who received the pentavalent vaccine and 45 million infants who received DTP. They calculated the risk of death within 72 hours after receipt of the pentavalent vaccine compared to DTP vaccination.

- There were 4.8 deaths per million vaccinated with DTP and 9.6 deaths per million vaccinated with pentavalent vaccine (odds ratio, OR = 1.98).

- Twice as many babies died shortly after receiving a pentavalent vaccine compared to babies vaccinated with DTP.

- Not all deaths following vaccination occur within 72 hours, so the findings in this paper are likely to have underestimated total deaths.

- If data from regions of India with better reporting of adverse events are projected nationally, the vaccine might cause more than 7000 deaths annually.

- Vietnam suspended use of the pentavalent vaccine after it caused 9 deaths. The World Health Organization (WHO) investigated the deaths and claimed that this vaccine was never associated with fatalities. But WHO had previously investigated similar deaths in Sri Lanka with no alternate explanation.

Influenza

The studies in this chapter cover a wide range of topics surrounding the detrimental effects of the influenza vaccine. For example, vaccinating pregnant women against influenza to protect their babies is not effective, and women vaccinated in their first trimester of pregnancy had high rates of spontaneous abortion. One study found that influenza vaccination during pregnancy may increase the risk of autism.

Several studies found that the influenza vaccine is not effective in infants or teenagers. It also increases the risk of contracting a respiratory illness caused by a non-influenza pathogen. Vaccinated elderly people are more likely to develop influenza than unvaccinated elderly people. Several studies show that vaccines grown in chicken eggs mutate as it adapts to the egg-based production process, leading to poor vaccine effectiveness.

Influenza vaccine effectiveness is influenced by the time of day the vaccine is administered, and also by the recipients mood on the day of vaccination. Additionally, the influenza vaccine increases the risk of developing non-Hodgkin lymphoma and of contracting a coronavirus infection. These are just some of the studies in this chapter that make the influenza vaccine problematic.

9.

It is unethical to mandate influenza vaccines for healthcare workers without reliable evidence of benefit to patients

"We conclude that policies of enforced influenza vaccination of healthcare workers to reduce patient risk lack a sound empirical basis. In that context, an intuitive sense that there may be some evidence in support of some patient benefit is insufficient scientific basis to ethically override individual healthcare worker rights."

De Serres G, Skowronski DM, et al. **Influenza vaccination of healthcare workers: critical analysis of the evidence for patient benefit underpinning policies of enforcement.** *PloS One* 2017 Jan 27; 12(1): e0163586.

- Health authorities rely on four studies to justify mandating influenza vaccines for healthcare workers to protect their patients. In this paper, scientists analyzed these studies for reliability of evidence supporting these policies.

- All of the studies greatly overestimated indirect patient benefit attributable to increased influenza vaccine coverage of healthcare workers.

- When the findings in the four studies are extrapolated to all hospital staff in the United States, an implausible 675,000 patient deaths would be prevented annually — exceeding estimated mortality during the 1918 pandemic.

- Analysis of actual patient data shows that 6,000 to 32,000 healthcare workers would need to be vaccinated to prevent one patient death. The belief that unvaccinated workers put their patients in great jeopardy is exaggerated.

- Proponents of mandatory vaccination have an obligation to ensure that the evidence they cite to justify health-related policies is trustworthy.

- A coherent influenza prevention program would require *all* healthcare workers, vaccinated or unvaccinated, to wear masks since more than 40% of *vaccinated* healthcare workers remain susceptible to influenza.

- Current scientific evidence does not support mandating influenza vaccination or healthcare workers to protect their patients.

10.

Influenza-vaccinated pregnant women weren't able to protect their babies and had high rates of spontaneous abortions

"We did not observe any reduction in rates of influenza or pneumonia among infants born to mothers who had received the monovalent pandemic vaccine during pregnancy compared with non-exposed infants."

Fell DB, Wilson K, et al. **Infant respiratory outcomes associated with prenatal exposure to maternal 2009 A/H1N1 influenza vaccination.** PloS One 2016 Aug 3; 11(8): e0160342.

- This study assessed whether influenza vaccination during pregnancy affects rates of infant influenza and pneumonia.

- Researchers analyzed 117,335 infant records. There were no differences in rates of influenza or pneumonia among infants born to influenza-vaccinated mothers compared with infants whose mothers were influenza-unvaccinated.

11.

Donahue JG, Kieke BA, et al. **Association of spontaneous abortion with receipt of inactivated influenza vaccine containing H1N1pdm09 in 2010-11 and 2011-12.** *Vaccine* 2017 Sep 25; 35(40): 5314-22.

"Spontaneous abortion was associated with influenza vaccination in the preceding 28 days."

- This study determined if vaccinating pregnant women against influenza in the first trimester is associated with spontaneous abortion (miscarriage).

- Women who had a spontaneous abortion were twice as likely to have received an influenza vaccine within the previous 28 days when compared to women who had full-term pregnancies (adjusted odds ratio, aOR = 2.0).

- Women who had a miscarriage were nearly 8 times more likely to have received an influenza vaccine in the current year and an H1N1/influenza vaccine in the previous year, compared to women without miscarriages (aOR = 7.7).

12.

Influenza vaccination during pregnancy may increase the risk of autism

"There was a suggestion of increased autism spectrum disorder risk among children whose mothers received an influenza vaccination in their first trimester, but the association was not statistically significant after adjusting for multiple comparisons, indicating that the finding could be due to chance."

Zerbo O, Qian Y, et al. **Association between influenza infection and vaccination during pregnancy and risk of autism spectrum disorder.** *JAMA Pediatr* 2017 Jan 2; 171(1): e163609.

- Influenza infection and influenza vaccination are associated with immune activation. Animal studies show a link between immune activation during pregnancy and autistic-like behavioral and brain disorders in offspring.

- This study was designed to determine whether pregnant women who become infected with influenza or receive an influenza vaccine have an increased risk of children with autism.

- There was no association between influenza infection during pregnancy and risk of autism. However, maternal influenza vaccination in the first trimester was associated with a statistically significant increased risk of children with autism (adjusted hazard ratio, AHR = 1.20).

- After adjusting for the multiplicity of hypotheses tested (using the Bonferroni correction), the authors concluded that the results could be due to chance.

- Use of the Bonferroni correction may be inappropriate because the associations were highly interdependent and the original findings may be real. [Hooker BS. *JAMA Pediatr* 2017 Apr 24.]

- The authors of this paper believe that additional studies are warranted to further evaluate any potential links between first-trimester maternal influenza vaccination and autism.

13.

A child's first exposure to influenza provides lifelong protective benefits against all similar strains of influenza

"Our findings show that major patterns in zoonotic influenza A virus epidemiology, previously attributed to patient age, are in fact driven by birth year. Influenza A virus strains circulating during an individual's childhood confer long-term protection against novel hemagglutinin subtypes from the same phylogenetic group. Hence, antigenic seniority extends across influenza A virus subtypes, introducing previously unrecognized generational structure to influenza epidemiology."

Gostic KM, Ambrose M, et al. **Potent protection against H5N1 and H7N9 influenza via childhood hemagglutinin imprinting.** *Science* 2016 Nov 11; 354(6313): 722-26.

- Two influenza A viruses of global concern severely infect different age groups. H5N1 causes extreme illness in younger people while H7N9 is more dangerous in older cohorts. Study authors sought to explain these puzzling differences.

- Influenza viruses contain hemagglutinin (HA), which influences susceptibility to influenza. HA subtypes H1, H2, and H5 are in the same phylogenetic group; subtypes H3 and H7 belong to a different phylogenetic group.

- In this paper, the authors show that children imprint on the HA group of their first exposure to influenza A, gaining future protection against severe illness from novel (pandemic) influenza A viruses within the same group.

- From 1918-1968, most children were initially exposed to H1 and H2 subtypes, protecting them in later life against severe illness from H5N1. Since 1968, most children were initially exposed to H3, conferring immunity against H7N9.

- Cross-protection gained from previous exposure to related pathogens benefits the individual and contributes substantially to natural herd immunity.

- These findings raise concerns that influenza vaccines given to children might prevent phylogenetic group imprinting from natural influenza infection, impairing natural long-term protection against emerging pandemic strains.

14.

The influenza vaccine is not effective in infants or adolescents

"Our conclusion is that influenza vaccination should not be strongly recommended for 6- to 11-month-old children."

Sugaya N, Shinjoh M, et al. **Three-season effectiveness of inactivated influenza vaccine in preventing influenza illness and hospitalization in children in Japan, 2013-2016.** *Vaccine* 2018 Feb 14; 36(8): 1063-1071.

- Scientists assessed influenza vaccine effectiveness in children 6 months to 15 years of age during three influenza seasons, from 2013 through 2016.

- The influenza vaccine was not effective in infants and provided low or non-significant effectiveness in 13- to 15-year-old adolescents.

15.

Sugaya N, Shinjoh M, et al. **Trivalent inactivated influenza vaccine effective against influenza A(H3N2) variant viruses in children during the 2014/15 season, Japan.** *Euro Surveill* 2016 Oct 20; 21(42): 30377.

- In this study, scientists assessed influenza vaccine effectiveness in children 6 months to 15 years of age during the 2014/15 influenza season.

- The influenza vaccine was found to be -5% (negative 5%) effective in infants. (Vaccinated infants were more likely than unvaccinated infants to develop the disease.) The vaccine was not effective in 13- to 15-year-old adolescents.

16.

Jackson ML, Chung JR, et al. **Influenza vaccine effectiveness in the United States during the 2015-2016 season.** *N Engl J Med* 2017 Aug 10; 377(6): 534-43.

- The influenza vaccine was found to be -19% (negative 19%) effective in children 2 to 17 years of age against laboratory-confirmed influenza. (Vaccinated children were more likely than unvaccinated children to develop the disease.)

17.

Influenza vaccination increases the risk of contracting a respiratory illness caused by a non-influenza pathogen

"Patients' experiences of increased respiratory illness after influenza vaccination may be supported by our finding of an increased rate of laboratory-confirmed non-influenza respiratory infections in the 14 days following vaccination."

Rikin S, Jia H, et al. **Assessment of temporally-related acute respiratory illness following influenza vaccination.** *Vaccine* 2018 Apr 5; 36(15): 1958-64.

• Researchers monitored 999 vaccinated and unvaccinated individuals over 3 influenza seasons to compare their rates of respiratory illness.

• Vaccinated children were significantly more likely than non-vaccinated children to contract non-influenza respiratory illness (hazard ratio, HR = 2.02 in a sensitivity analysis).

18.

Dierig A, Heron LG, et al. **Epidemiology of respiratory viral infections in children enrolled in a study of influenza vaccine effectiveness.** *Influenza Other Respir Viruses* 2014 May; 8(3): 293-301.

"Recipients of influenza vaccines had about 1.6 times more influenza-like illness episodes than did unvaccinated children. It should be a priority to determine whether...any observed increase in the rate of non-influenza respiratory virus identification outweighs the benefit of seasonal trivalent influenza vaccines in children."

• In this study, 381 children 6-35 months of age were classified as either fully vaccinated (2 doses), partially vaccinated (1 dose), or unvaccinated against influenza. They were then monitored for cases for influenza-like illness.

• Influenza-like illness was significantly more common in fully and partially vaccinated children than among unvaccinated subjects (rate ratio, RR = 1.6).

19.

Doctor visits for preventive care increase the risk of subsequent doctor visits for influenza-like illness

"Our results demonstrate that well-child visits are associated with influenza-like illness visits during the week of and two weeks following a well-child visit."

Simmering JE, Polgreen LA, et al. **Are well-child visits a risk factor for subsequent influenza-like illness visits?** *Infect Control Hosp Epidemiol* 2014 Mar; 35(3): 251-56.

- In doctors' waiting rooms, young children with respiratory infections may spread disease to healthy children and their parents.

- During a 13-year study period, researchers analyzed medical data on 84,595 U.S. families to determine if well-child visits (preventive healthcare) increase the risk of subsequent influenza-like illness within the child's family.

- Influenza-like illnesses include diagnoses of influenza, pneumonia, bronchitis, pharyngitis, viral infections, and upper respiratory disease.

- This study found that when a family member developed an influenza-like illness the likelihood of a well-child visit in the same week, or within the previous two weeks, was significantly increased (odds ratio, OR = 1.54).

- For every well-child visit, there was a 3.17% increased probability that a family member would develop an influenza-like illness within the following two weeks.

- The additional risk of developing an influenza-like illness within the following two weeks of a well-child visit translates to approximately 778,974 excess cases per year with an economic burden greater than $500 million annually.

- This study did not examine the possibility that some cases of influenza-like illness that occurred in family members within the following two weeks of a well-child visit may have been related to vaccines received by the child.

20.

The live attenuated influenza vaccine induces rapid proliferation of pathogenic bacteria capable of causing severe disease

"Here we show, in mice, that vaccination with live attenuated influenza primes the upper respiratory tract for increased bacterial growth and persistence of bacterial carriage, in a manner nearly identical to that seen following wild-type influenza virus infections."

Mina MJ, McCullers JA, Klugman KP. **Live attenuated influenza vaccine enhances colonization of** *Streptococcus pneumoniae* **and** *Staphylococcus aureus* **in mice.** *Mbio* 2014 Feb 18; 5(1): e01040-13.

- Infection with wild influenza viruses increases susceptibility to bacterial pathogens that are a primary cause of pneumonia, bacteremia, and flu-related mortality. This study was designed to determine whether similar effects occur following receipt of a live attenuated influenza vaccine (LAIV).

- In this study, scientists vaccinated groups of mice with either LAIV (adapted for mice from the human FluMist vaccine), a wild-type influenza virus, or placebo. They then analyzed and compared bacterial dynamics within the nasal cavities/nasopharynx of the mice.

- This study found that vaccination with LAIV reverses normal bacterial clearance from the nasopharynx and significantly increases upper respiratory tract densities of bacterial pathogen strains associated with severe morbidity and mortality (*Streptococcus pneumoniae* and *Staphylococcus aureus*).

- Within 3 days post-vaccination, pathogenic bacteria exhibited exponential growth and extended the mean duration of colonization from 35 to 57 days, effects similar to those induced by a wild-type influenza infection.

- Mice infected with pneumococcus 28 days post-vaccination had up to 4-fold increases in excess bacterial proliferation compared to unvaccinated controls.

- Live attenuated viral vaccines may have unintended consequences associated with the acquisition, colonization, and transmission/spread of severe disease-causing bacterial pathogens unrelated to those targeted by the vaccine.

21.

Vaccinated elderly people are more likely to develop influenza than unvaccinated elderly people

"In the study population, vaccine effectiveness against laboratory-confirmed influenza A was -11% [minus 11%]."

Bragstad K, Emborg H, et al. **Low vaccine effectiveness against influenza A(H3N2) virus among elderly people in Denmark in 2012/13—a rapid epidemiological and virological assessment.** *Euro Surveill* 2013 Feb 7; 18(6): 20397.

- In this study, scientists calculated influenza vaccine effectiveness among elderly people in Denmark during the 2012/13 influenza season.

- The vaccine was -11% (negative 11%) effective against laboratory-confirmed influenza A. (Vaccinated people were more likely than unvaccinated people to develop the disease.)

22.

Pebody R, Warburton F, et al. **End-of-season influenza vaccine effectiveness in adults and children, United Kingdom, 2016-17.** *Euro Surveill* 2017 Nov 2; 22(44): 17-00306.

- Public health officials in England reported that the influenza vaccine was -68% (negative 68%) effective in the elderly population against the virulent influenza A(H3N2) strain during the 2016/17 influenza season. (Vaccinated people were more likely than unvaccinated people to develop the disease.)

23.

Influenza vaccines grown in chicken eggs mutate during vaccine production causing poor effectiveness

"While evolutionary drift in circulating viruses cannot be regulated, mutations that are introduced as part of egg-based vaccine production may be amenable to improvements."

Skowronski DM, Janjua NZ, et al. **Low 2012-13 influenza vaccine effectiveness associated with mutation in the egg-adapted H3N2 vaccine strain not antigenic drift in circulating viruses.** *PloS One* 2014 Mar 25; 9(3): e92153.

- Health experts have historically known that a mismatch between influenza vaccine composition and circulating viruses (due to evolutionary drift) would result in low vaccine effectiveness. Conversely, they thought that a perfect match would ensure good protection.

- During a recent influenza epidemic in Canada and elsewhere globally, the influenza vaccine did not provide adequate protection despite an identical match between the circulating virus and the prototype virus recommended for vaccine production by the World Health Organization.

- In this paper, Canadian scientists conducted epidemiological and laboratory investigations to understand why influenza vaccine effectiveness is low even during years when there is a perfect match between vaccine composition and circulating viruses.

- Detailed gene sequencing and hemagglutinin analyses revealed that poor vaccine protection was due to mutations in the egg-adapted influenza vaccine strain during vaccine production, not antigenic drift in circulating viruses.

- This study shows that a perfect match between circulating influenza viruses and the influenza viruses recommended for vaccine production by the World Health Organization cannot ensure adequate vaccine effectiveness because the vaccine strain can mutate during vaccine production.

24.

Influenza vaccines grown in chicken eggs target the egg-adapted vaccine strain, not the wild strain in society

"The effectiveness of the annual influenza vaccine has declined in recent years. A major cause for this lack in effectiveness has been attributed to the egg-based vaccine production process."

Wu NC, Zost SJ, et al. **A structural explanation for the low effectiveness of the seasonal influenza H3N2 vaccine.** *PloS Pathog* 2017 Oct 23; 13(10): e1006682.

- People who are vaccinated against influenza are not always protected because an influenza virus grown in chicken eggs often mutates as it adapts to the egg-based vaccine production process, resulting in poor vaccine effectiveness.

25.

Raymond DD, Stewart SM, et al. **Influenza immunization elicits antibodies specific for an egg-adapted vaccine strain.** *Nat Med* 2016 Dec; 22(12): 1465-69.

"The most notable conclusion from this study is that many vaccine-elicited antibodies fail to bind or neutralize the corresponding circulating strain because of their specificity for a mutation that adapted the vaccine strain for growth in chicken eggs."

- Influenza vaccines grown in chicken eggs induce antibodies that recognize the egg-adapted vaccine strain, not the wild strain circulating in society.

26.

Chen Z, Zhou H, Jin H. **The impact of key amino acid substitutions in the hemagglutinin of influenza A (H3N2) viruses on vaccine production and antibody response.** *Vaccine* 2010 May 28; 28(24): 4079-85.

- Vaccines produced in eggs may fail to elicit a protective immune response.

27.

Scientists knew that influenza vaccines grown in chicken eggs induce antigenic changes rendering the vaccine ineffective

"Our findings demonstrate the capacity for a single amino acid change in the hemagglutinin to markedly influence the immune recognition of influenza virus."

Kodihalli S, Justewicz DM, et al. **Selection of a single amino acid substitution in the hemagglutinin molecule by chicken eggs can render influenza A virus (H3) candidate vaccine ineffective.** *J Virol* 1995 Aug; 69(8): 4888-97.

• Embryonated chicken eggs provide an inexpensive way to mass produce influenza vaccines quickly. However, evidence has shown that the medium in which the virus is cultivated can induce antigenic variations of concern.

• In this study, scientists investigated whether a single amino acid change in the hemagglutinin molecule during influenza vaccine production in embryonated chicken eggs can influence vaccine efficacy.

• Study results show that a) some of the hemagglutinin variations that occur during passage in eggs are sufficiently different from influenza viruses that cause clinical disease, and b) they induce post-vaccination antibody responses to influenza that are clinically irrelevant.

28.

Robertson JS, Bootman JS, et al. **Structural changes in the haemagglutinin which accompany egg adaptation of an influenza A(H1N1) virus.** *Virology* 1987 Sep; 160(1): 31-37.

"Antigenic changes are often induced in the haemagglutinin of human isolates of influenza A and B viruses during their isolation and propagation in embryonated hens' eggs. In this study, at least three antigenically distinct groups of egg-adapted variants were observed. These observations have implications for the indiscriminate use of egg-adapted viruses in seroepidemiological studies and vaccine production."

29.

Influenza vaccine effectiveness depends on the time of day the vaccine is given and mood of the recipient

"Adjusting the timing of vaccination may be a simple, cost neutral and effective public health intervention to improve vaccination responses, particularly in older adults. However, it is possible that the best time of day for vaccination may be different for different vaccines."

Long JE, Drayson MT, et al. **Morning vaccination enhances antibody response over afternoon vaccination: a cluster-randomised trial.** *Vaccine* 2016 May 23; 34(24): 2679-85.

- In this study, 276 adults aged 65 years or older were either vaccinated in the morning (9-11am) or afternoon (3-5pm). One month later, their vaccine-induced antibody levels were measured. Influenza vaccination in the morning was associated with a significantly greater antibody response ($p = .05$).

30.

Ayling K, Fairclough L, et al. **Positive mood on the day of influenza vaccination predicts vaccine effectiveness: A prospective observational cohort study.** *Brain Behav Immun* 2018 Jan; 67: 314-23.

"Greater positive mood in older adults, particularly on the day of vaccination, is associated with enhanced responses to vaccination."

- In this study, 138 adults (65 to 85 years of age) had data collected daily for 6 weeks quantifying physical activity levels, dietary intake, sleep duration, stress levels, and emotional affect (positive or negative mood).

- A positive mood on the day of vaccination was significantly predictive of higher IgG levels at 4 weeks ($r = 0.26$) and 16 weeks ($r = 0.35$) post-vaccination.

- There also was a significant relationship between having a positive mood during the 6-week data collection period and higher antibody levels at 4 weeks ($r = 0.20$) and 16 weeks ($r = 0.30$) post-vaccination.

31.

Aspirin therapy during the 1918-1919 influenza pandemic might have contributed to high mortality

"Just before the 1918 death spike, aspirin was recommended in regimens now known to be potentially toxic and to cause pulmonary edema and may therefore have contributed to overall pandemic mortality."

Starko KM. **Salicylates and pandemic influenza mortality, 1918-1919 pharmacology, pathology, and historic evidence.** *Clin Infect Dis* 2009 Nov 1; 49(9): 1405-10.

- During the "Spanish influenza" pandemic, deaths in the United States peaked with a sudden spike in October 1918. The author of this paper provides evidence that a significant proportion of the deaths may be attributed to the recommended use of aspirin to treat influenza.

- The big death spike in October 1918 occurred shortly after the Surgeon General of the Unites States Army (Sep 13), the U.S. Navy (Sep 26) and the *Journal of the American Medical Association* (Oct 5) all recommended very large daily doses of aspirin to treat influenza.

- In 1918, doctors recommended 1000-1300 mg of aspirin (as acetylsalicylic acid or sodium salicylate) in frequencies ranging from hourly to every 3 hours, resulting in daily doses of 8-31 grams, well above toxicity levels. (Progressive salicylate toxicity was indistinguishable from pathological infection.)

- Pulmonary edema in humans with salicylate intoxication is well documented. Salicylates increase lung fluid and impair the body's ability to clear mucus from the respiratory tract. In one study, pulmonary edema was found at autopsy in 46% of 26 salicylate-intoxicated adults.

- The military's regimented use of aspirin therapy likely contributed to the pandemic's high mortality rate in young adults.

- From the 1950s to the 1980s, thousands of deaths following influenza and other viral infections were unexplained until studies identified aspirin as the major contributor to Reye syndrome toxicity.

32.

Influenza vaccines significantly increase the risk of developing non-Hodgkin lymphoma

"We found that ever receiving an influenza vaccine was associated with a higher risk of non-Hodgkin lymphoma."

Lankes HA, Fought AJ, et al. **Vaccination history and risk of non-Hodgkin lymphoma: a population-based, case-control study.** *Cancer Causes Control* 2009 Jul; 20(5): 517-23.

- Non-Hodgkin lymphoma (NHL) is a type of cancer that develops in white blood cells called lymphocytes, which are part of the body's immune system.

- Since autoimmune disorders and chronic infections can increase the risk of NHL, it is plausible that vaccinations, which are designed to induce immune responses, may also be associated with NHL risk.

- In this study, tetanus, polio, influenza, smallpox, and tuberculosis vaccine histories of 387 patients with NHL were compared to 535 controls.

- A history of influenza vaccination was associated with a significantly higher risk of developing non-Hodgkin lymphoma (odds ratio, OR = 1.53).

- This study also explored whether vaccinations affect the development of NHL subtypes. A history of influenza vaccination was associated with a nearly twofold higher risk of developing follicular lymphoma (OR = 1.98) and diffuse large B cell lymphoma (OR = 1.88).

- Ever having received an influenza vaccine was associated with a significantly increased risk of both low grade and high grade lymphoma.

- NHL risk was found to be inversely associated with ever having received a polio or smallpox vaccine.

- Risk patterns were similar in men and women.

33.

Vaccination against influenza significantly increases the risk of contracting a coronavirus infection

"Vaccinated individuals may be at increased risk for other respiratory viruses because they do not receive the non-specific immunity associated with natural infection."

Wolff GG. **Influenza vaccination and respiratory virus interference among Department of Defense personnel during the 2017-2018 influenza season.** *Vaccine* 2020 Jan 10; 38(2): 350-54.

- Recent evidence suggests that natural influenza infections may provide cross protection against non-influenza viral infections. In contrast, influenza-vaccinated people do not receive this non-specific immunity and may be at increased risk for other respiratory viruses.

- This study, conducted during the 2017-2018 influenza season, investigated whether vaccination against influenza increases the risk of contracting other non-influenza respiratory viruses, a phenomenon known as virus interference.

- The study population consisted of 9469 U.S. active duty service members 18-35 years of age.

- This study found that influenza-vaccinated individuals had a reduced risk of developing influenza but were significantly more likely than unvaccinated people to contract a coronavirus infection (odds ratio, OR = 1.36; $p < 0.01$).

- Influenza-vaccinated individuals were also more likely to develop human metapneumovirus (OR = 1.51).

Influenza and Annual Vaccinations

The policy of recommending annual influenza vaccinations has been questioned by field studies since the 1970s when data showed a loss of protective immunity following repeated vaccinations. Hoskins found that the influenza vaccine was only effective in individuals who were vaccinated for the first time with the most up-to-date strain. Numerous studies continue to confirm that influenza vaccination during prior years may reduce vaccine effectiveness (VE) in the current year.

Skowronski (2016) found that influenza VE against A(H3N2) — the predominant circulating strain during the season under analysis — was 53%. However, if patients were also vaccinated in the prior year, VE was significantly lower at -32%. VE was -54% for patients who were also vaccinated in previous two years. (People vaccinated 3 years in a row were 54% more likely than unvaccinated people to contract a severe case of influenza requiring medical attention.) In Italy, Rizzo found that influenza vaccine recipients (who were also mostly repeat influenza vaccine recipients during previous years) were 85% more likely than non-vaccinated people to contract influenza (-84.5%; 95% CI, -190.4 to -17.2%).

Scientists can explain why influenza vaccination during prior years reduces VE in the current year. According to the *antigenic distance* hypothesis, repeated vaccination can reduce VE when a) the prior season and current season vaccines are antigenically similar to each other, and b) the current season circulating virus has drifted. If antibodies from a prior influenza vaccine are high for more than a year, they can cause negative interference (or a negative antigenic interaction) with a new influenza vaccine. According to Smith, skipping vaccination for a year is one possible way to avoid this effect in the following year. If there is a choice, health officials should choose a vaccine strain most unlike the previous vaccine strain to avoid negative interference in repeat vaccinees.

34.

Influenza vaccination during prior years reduces vaccine effectiveness in the current year

"This study raises relevant questions about the potential interference of repeated annual influenza vaccination."

McLean HQ, Thompson MG, et al. **Impact of repeated vaccination on vaccine effectiveness against influenza A(H3N2) and B during 8 seasons.** *Clin Infect Dis* 2014 Nov 15; 59(10): 1375-85.

- Several studies have shown that influenza vaccine effectiveness in the current season is significantly reduced in people who also received an influenza vaccine during the previous year.

- In this study of 7,315 people with acute respiratory infection, researchers assessed influenza vaccine effectiveness in the current season in people that were either unvaccinated or vaccinated 1-5 times during the prior 5 influenza seasons.

- Cases were people with laboratory confirmed influenza; controls tested negative for influenza.

- Study results show that current-season influenza vaccine effectiveness was significantly higher among vaccinated people who did not receive an influenza vaccine during the previous 5 years compared with vaccinated people who were frequently vaccinated during the same period (65% vs 24%; $p = .01$).

- Current year vaccine effectiveness was 65%, 35%, and 24% in people who were unvaccinated, vaccinated 1-3 times, or vaccinated 4-5 times during the previous 5 years, respectively.

- Influenza vaccine-induced protection was significantly diminished in people who received influenza vaccines during the prior 5 years.

- The authors speculate that "vaccine interference" may be occurring due to original antigenic sin, immune exhaustion, and/or antigenic drift of circulating influenza viruses in relation to vaccine antigens.

35.

People vaccinated in successive influenza seasons were significantly more likely than unvaccinated people to contract influenza

"Variation in the viral genome and negative effects of serial vaccination likely contributed to poor influenza vaccine performance."

Skowronski DM, Chambers C, et al. **A perfect storm: impact of genomic variation and serial vaccination on low influenza vaccine effectiveness during the 2014-2015 season.** *Clin Infect Dis* 2016 Jul 1; 63(1): 21-32.

- This study measured the effects of prior-year influenza vaccinations on influenza vaccine effectiveness (VE) in the current year.

- In the 2014-15 influenza season, overall VE against the predominant A(H3N2) subtype of laboratory-confirmed influenza was -17% (negative 17%). Vaccine effectiveness was -64% (negative 64%) in children 1-19 years of age.

- For patients vaccinated against influenza in the current year but not in earlier years, the vaccine was 53% effective. However, if they were also vaccinated in the prior year, VE was significantly lower at -32% (negative 32%).

- VE was -54% for patients who were also vaccinated in the previous 2 years. (People vaccinated 3 years in a row were 54% more likely than unvaccinated people to contract a severe case of influenza requiring medical attention.)

- Negative interference from prior influenza vaccination occurs when vaccine strains are similar in successive years but mismatched to the circulating virus.

36.

Rizzo C, Bella A, et al. **Influenza vaccine effectiveness in Italy: age, subtype-specific and vaccine type estimates 2014/15 season.** *Vaccine* 2016 Jun 8; 34(27): 3102-08.

- In Italy, influenza vaccine recipients in 2014-15 (who were also mostly repeat influenza vaccine recipients during previous seasons) were significantly more likely than unvaccinated people to contract influenza A(H3N2) (OR = 1.85).

37.

Influenza vaccination two years in a row increases the risk of contracting influenza

"Repeat vaccine recipients over two seasons had a significantly 2-fold higher risk of A(H1N1) illness than participants vaccinated during the current season only."

Skowronski DM, Chambers C, et al. **Beyond antigenic match: possible agent-host and immuno-epidemiological influences on influenza vaccine effectiveness during the 2015-2016 season in Canada.** *J Infect Dis* 2017 Dec 19; 216(12): 1487-1500.

- This study assessed factors that influence influenza vaccine effectiveness, such as within-season waning of protection and prior-year vaccination.

- People who received an influenza vaccine in two consecutive years were twice as likely to contract influenza compared with those who received an influenza vaccine in the current year only (odds ratio, OR = 2.33).

- This study confirmed statistically significant negative interference by a prior-year influenza vaccine on the current year's vaccine effectiveness.

38.

Ohmit SE, Thompson MG, et al. **Influenza vaccine effectiveness in the 2011-2012 season: protection against each circulating virus and the effect of prior vaccination on estimates.** *Clin Infect Dis* 2014 Feb; 58(3): 319-27.

"We also demonstrated an apparent negative effect of repeated annual vaccination on effectiveness."

- In this study of 4,771 individuals, the vaccine offered no significant protection in people who were also vaccinated in the prior season.

- Children under nine years of age were enrolled in the overall study, but they were excluded from an analysis of the potential negative effect of prior year vaccination on current year vaccine effectiveness.

39.

The current season's influenza vaccine is less effective in people who were also vaccinated in the prior season

"Lower vaccine effectiveness was observed in those vaccinated in both the current and prior seasons, compared with those vaccinated in the current season only."

Ohmit SE, Petrie JG, et al. **Influenza vaccine effectiveness in households with children during the 2012-2013 season: assessments of prior vaccination and serologic susceptibility.** *J Infect Dis* 2015 May 15; 211(10): 1519-28.

- The current-year vaccine was less effective in individuals who were also vaccinated in the prior year.

- In children under 9 years of age, the risk of developing influenza was higher in those who were *fully* vaccinated rather than *partially* vaccinated.

40.

Shinjoh M, Sugaya N, et al. **Inactivated influenza vaccine effectiveness and an analysis of repeated vaccination for children during the 2016/17 season.** *Vaccine* 2018 Sep 5; 36(37): 5510-18.

"We have shown that influenza vaccination was effective only when children were vaccinated in the current season."

- Children who were vaccinated in two seasons — both last year and during the current year — were significantly more likely to develop influenza compared to those who were vaccinated in the current season only (AOR = 1.53).

- The vaccine provided no benefit to infants. The authors conclude that influenza vaccination should not be strongly recommended for 6- to 11-month-old babies.

- Children who contracted a wild influenza infection in the previous season are likely to acquire strong immunity against influenza in the current season.

41.

People vaccinated against influenza two seasons in a row are 6 times more infectious than unvaccinated people

"Vaccination for the current season was associated with a trend toward higher viral shedding; vaccination with both the current and previous year's seasonal vaccines was significantly associated with greater fine-aerosol shedding. We observed 6.3 times more aerosol shedding among cases with vaccination in the current and previous season compared with having no vaccination in those two seasons."

Yan J, Grantham M, et al. **Infectious virus in exhaled breath of sympto-matic seasonal influenza cases from a college community.** *Proc Natl Acad Sci USA* 2018 Jan 30; 115(5): 1081-86.

- This study was designed to identify factors that impact airborne influenza transmission. Scientists measured the aerosol infectiousness (viral shedding capacity) of breathing, talking, coughing, and sneezing in 142 college students with confirmed influenza infection.

- Cough frequency was significantly associated with increased fine- and coarse-aerosol shedding. Fine-aerosol shedding was significantly greater for males. On average, males produced 3.2 times more virus than did females per cough. However, females coughed significantly more frequently than males.

- Although coughing was prevalent with influenza infection and a strong predictor of viral shedding, it's not required to generate aerosol infectiousness.

- Influenza symptoms were not significant predictors for aerosol shedding.

- Individuals who received seasonal influenza vaccines in the current and previous seasons had 6.3 times more aerosol shedding when compared with individuals who were not vaccinated in those two seasons.

- Influenza vaccination during the current and prior year was associated with a significant increase in shedding of the influenza A virus. In combination with recent literature suggesting reduced protection with annual vaccination, influenza vaccine recommendations and policies may need to be reassessed.

42.

Children who are influenza-vaccinated in the current and previous seasons have worse outcomes than unvaccinated children

"Little or no vaccine protection was observed overall, with adjusted vaccine effectiveness against medically attended influenza A(H3N2) infection of negative 8%. Given these findings, other adjunct measures should be considered."

Skowronski DM, Chambers C, et al. **Interim estimates of 2014/15 vaccine effectiveness against influenza A(H3N2) from Canada's Sentinel Physician Surveillance Network, January 2015.** *Euro Surveil* 2015 Jan 29; 20(4): 21022.

- This study evaluated influenza vaccine effectiveness (VE) in Canada for 12 weeks during the 2014/2015 influenza season.

- Unadjusted VE (in all age groups) against the predominant circulating influenza A(H3N2) strain was negative 21% but improved to negative 8% after adjusting for covariates.

- VE against influenza A(H3N2) was 43% among those who were vaccinated in the current year (but not in the previous year). If they were also vaccinated in the previous year, VE was significantly lower at negative 15%.

- Vaccinated children (up to 19 years of age) were more than twice as likely to develop a severe case of influenza compared to unvaccinated children (crude odds ratio, OR = 2.18, calculated from Table 3A).

- Vaccinated children (1 to 8 years of age) were nearly 3 times as likely to develop a severe case of influenza (requiring medical attention) compared to unvaccinated children (crude odds ratio, OR = 2.66).

- Negative VE could be attributed to 1) a mismatch between vaccine viruses and genetically distinct circulating viruses, and 2) negative interference from prior vaccination, consistent with the antigenic distance hypothesis.

43.

Annual influenza vaccinations increase the odds of developing a severe case of influenza

"Effects of repeat influenza vaccination were consistent with the antigenic distance hypothesis and may have contributed to findings of low vaccine effectiveness across recent A(H3N2) epidemics."

Skowronski DM, Chambers C, et al. **Serial vaccination and the antigenic distance hypothesis: effects on influenza vaccine effectiveness during A(H3N2) epidemics in Canada, 2010-2011 to 2014-2015.** *J Infect Dis* 2017 Apr 1; 215(7): 1059-99.

- The "antigenic distance hypothesis" (ADH) explains why a current year's influenza vaccine often is less effective when the recipient was also vaccinated in a prior year. This negative effect occurs when the previous and current vaccines are antigenically similar and the circulating virus has drifted.

- In this study, scientists tested the ADH against medically attended, laboratory-confirmed influenza by integrating two large clinical and virological databases to analyze how annual (repeat) influenza vaccinations may have contributed to poor vaccine effectiveness during 3 epidemics in Canada.

- During the 2010-11 influenza season, individuals who received an influenza vaccine during a prior season were significantly more likely to contract a severe case of influenza compared with people who were unvaccinated in the current and prior seasons (vaccine effectiveness = negative 55%).

- During the 2014-15 influenza season, individuals who received vaccines during the current and a prior season were nearly 4 times more likely to contract a severe case of influenza compared with those who only received an influenza vaccine in the current year (odds ratio, OR = 3.76).

- People who received vaccines during 2 prior seasons and the current season were significantly more likely to contract a severe case of influenza compared with those who were unvaccinated during all 3 seasons (OR = 1.47).

- Annual influenza vaccination is not associated with enhanced protection.

44.

Annual influenza vaccinations reduce protection against influenza

"Persistent antibodies were found in 71.9% of the group that had not received annual vaccinations and in 43.8% of the group that had received annual vaccinations."

Huijskens E, Rossen J, et al. **Immunogenicity, boostability, and sustainability of the immune response after vaccination against Influenza A virus (H1N1) 2009 in a healthy population.** *Clin Vaccine Immunol* 2011 Sep; 18(9): 1401-05.

- In this study, scientists measured immune responses in 498 healthcare workers before and after they were vaccinated against the influenza A virus.

- Humoral immunity was lower by 31% in adults with a history of annual influenza vaccination compared with adults not previously vaccinated.

45.

Beyer WE, Palache AM, et al. **Effects of repeated annual influenza vaccination on vaccine sero-response in young and elderly adults.** *Vaccine* 1996 Oct; 14(14): 1331-39.

"At a given pre-vaccination titre, the post-vaccination titre can be expected to be lower in previously vaccinated subjects than in not previously vaccinated subjects. The phenomenon could be described as a 'negative booster effect of previous vaccinations' suggesting an active immunological feedback mechanism which inhibits the production of additional post-vaccination antibody."

- Three studies conducted from 1986 to 1989 on 884 people provide evidence that post-vaccination antibody titers are strongly dependent, inversely, on the status of prior vaccination.

- The policy of recommending annual influenza vaccinations has been questioned by field studies since the 1970s when data showed a loss of protective immunity following repeated vaccinations.

46.

Immune protection from an influenza vaccine is compromised in people who also received a previous influenza vaccine

"Significantly fewer adults developed a presumably protective level of serum antibody to the new influenza A(H3N2) strain when they had been previously vaccinated."

Gross PA, Sperber SJ, et al. **Paradoxical response to a novel influenza virus vaccine strain: the effect of prior immunization.** *Vaccine* 1999 May 4; 17(18): 2284-89.

- In this randomized, double-blind study, researchers sought to determine if the immune response to a new influenza vaccine would be inferior in previously vaccinated people, compared with those not previously vaccinated.

- Previously vaccinated people had significantly lower post-vaccination antibody titers for all 3 strains in the new vaccine: A(H1N1), A(H3N2), and B.

- The percent of subjects with a presumed protective level of antibodies against the A(H3N2) strain was significantly lower in the previously vaccinated group.

- Subjects with a history of prior influenza vaccination had significantly higher antibody titers *before* receiving a new influenza vaccine but significantly lower titers *after* vaccination, compared to people not previously vaccinated.

47.

Sasaki S, He XS, et al. **Influence of prior influenza vaccination on antibody and B-cell responses.** *PloS One* 2008 Aug 20; 3(8): e2975.

"The efficacy of repeated vaccination...has been debated for many years. These data suggest that prior year vaccination with influenza vaccine...reduced the IgA effector B-cell response to new influenza immunization and may have a similar effect on the IgG B-cell response."

- Findings in this paper indicate that influenza vaccination in a prior year can lower serum antibody and B-cell responses to subsequent vaccination.

48.

Annual influenza vaccinations do not offer a special advantage over influenza vaccination for the first time

"Significant reductions in mean serum antibody levels and increased shedding of influenza A (H3N2) virus were noted with increasing numbers of annual immunizations during the last year of the study."

Keitel WA, Cate TR, et al. **Efficacy of repeated annual immunization with inactivated influenza virus vaccines over a five year period.** *Vaccine* 1997 Jul; 15(10): 1114-22.

• This study evaluated the efficacy of inactivated influenza vaccines over a 5-year period to determine whether they are less effective in people who receive them annually versus those receiving it for the first time.

• The risk of shedding influenza A (H3N2) virus was significantly increased with increasing numbers of annual vaccinations (OR = 1.48).

• Repeated vaccination did not appear to confer any special advantage over vaccination for the first time.

49.

Valenciano M, Kissling E, et al. **Vaccine effectiveness in preventing laboratory-confirmed influenza in primary care patients in a season of co-circulation of influenza A(H1N1)pdm09, B and drifted A(H3N2), I-MOVE Multicentre Case-Control Study, Europe 2014/15.** *Euro Surveill* 2016; 21(7): 30139.

"The efficacy of repeated vaccination...has been debated for many years."

• Scientists measured influenza vaccine effectiveness against laboratory-confirmed influenza in eight European countries.

• The vaccine was -5% (negative 5%) effective among people who were vaccinated during the current and previous influenza seasons.

51.

Scientists have known for many years that annual re-vaccination against influenza confers no long-term advantage

"The development of A/England/42/72 hemagglutinating antibody was less frequent after re-vaccination of boys in whom the A/Hong Kong/68 hemagglutinating antibody had been induced by vaccination."

Hoskins TW, Davies JR, et al. **Controlled trial of inactivated influenza vaccine containing the A/Hong Kong strain during an outbreak of influenza due to the A/England/42/72 strain.** *Lancet* 1973 Jul 21; 302(7821): 116-120.

- From 1970 to 1972, 800 boys in a boarding school had their antibodies measured. Some of the boys received an influenza vaccine containing the "Hong Kong" strain; the remaining boys were assigned to a control group.

- During an outbreak of influenza due to the "England" strain, most vaccinated boys who previously acquired natural immunity to the Hong Kong strain developed antibodies to the England strain. This occurred less often in boys with Hong Kong antibodies induced by prior vaccination.

52.

Hoskins, TW, Davies JR, et al. **Assessment of inactivated influenza-A vaccine after three outbreaks of influenza-A at Christ's Hospital.** *Lancet* 1979 Jan 6; 1(8106): 33-35.

"The cumulative attack-rate in the three outbreaks was similar in all groups irrespective of vaccination history. These observations suggest that annual re-vaccination with inactivated influenza-A vaccine confers no long-term advantage."

- During outbreaks of influenza in 1972, 1974, and 1976, the influenza vaccine was only effective in individuals who were vaccinated for the first time with the most up-to-date strain.

- The practice of annual influenza re-vaccination is questionable.

53.

The "antigenic distance hypothesis" predicts how and when annual influenza vaccines will reduce vaccine efficacy

"Our results show that antigenic distances between the first and second vaccines, and between the first vaccine and the epidemic strain, significantly affect [influenza] attack rates in repeat vaccinees."

Smith DJ, Forrest S, et al. **Variable efficacy of repeated annual influenza vaccination.** *Proc Natl Acad Sci USA* 1999 Nov 23; 96(24): 14001-14006.

- The authors of this paper developed a theory — the *antigenic distance* hypothesis — to explain variations in vaccine efficacy in people who receive more than one annual influenza vaccine.

- The *antigenic distance* hypothesis states that when people receive influenza vaccines with similar strains 2 years in a row, antibodies produced by the first vaccine cross-react with the new vaccine, inducing negative interference and a weak immune response.

- Positive interference occurs when strains in a previous influenza vaccine are antigenically similar to circulating strains in the current influenza season.

- Influenza vaccine efficacy depends on a combination of negative and positive interference induced by a previous influenza vaccine, influenced by the antigenic distance (degree of similarity) between a) the first and second vaccines, and b) the first vaccine and circulating strains in the current season.

- In this study, the antigenic distance hypothesis was tested on 7 influenza outbreaks and accurately predicted variations in vaccine efficacy in people who received one, or more than one, annual influenza vaccine.

- If antibodies from a prior vaccine are high for more than a year, they can negatively interfere with a new vaccine. Skipping vaccination for a year is one possible way to avoid negative interference in the following year.

- If there is a choice, health officials should choose a vaccine strain most unlike the previous vaccine strain to avoid negative interference in repeat vaccinees.

Influenza Vaccine and Guillain-Barré syndrome

Guillain-Barré syndrome (GBS) is a serious health condition in which a person's own immune system damages their nerve cells, causing muscle weakness and paralysis. About 30% of cases require tracheal intubation and mechanical ventilation to help with breathing and prevent respiratory failure. Often, there is difficulty with facial movements that affect the ability to eat, speak or swallow. Patients may be hospitalized for months and up to 10% will die.

About 20% of people afflicted with GBS are still incapacitated after 6 months and 30% have permanent or lifelong weakness. About 60% of those who require artificial ventilation will develop other medical problems such as pneumonia, severe infections, blood clots in the lungs and bleeding in the digestive tract. Following the acute phase, GBS patients often require months of intensive rehabilitation with a physical therapist, speech therapist, neurologist, psychologist, and other health professionals.

Although the precise etiology of GBS is unknown, it is often preceded by a gastrointestinal or respiratory infection. Vaccines are known to cause GBS as well. The studies in this chapter show significantly increased rates of GBS associated with 1) seasonal influenza vaccines, and 2) pandemic swine influenza vaccines (H1N1) administered during national vaccination campaigns in 1976-1977 and 2009-2010.

Since the median onset of GBS following influenza vaccination is approximately 2 weeks (with a range of 1-6 weeks), many of the studies were self-controlled comparisons of GBS rates 1-6 weeks post-vaccination versus 7-12 weeks post-vaccination. Often, the globally accepted Brighton Collaboration case definitions of GBS were utilized to provide diagnostic certainty. Findings in the studies indicate that influenza vaccination significantly increases the risk of GBS approximately 2 to 8 times (relative risk), and causes between 1 and 10 excess cases of GBS per million people vaccinated (attributable risk).

Seasonal influenza vaccines cause between 2 and 5 excess cases of GBS per million people vaccinated. These are cases of GBS directly attributable to the vaccine — above the normal baseline incidence of GBS. This may seem like a rare possibility. However, in the United States more than 140 million people are vaccinated against influenza annually. Thus, about 280 to 700 people may be stricken with GBS every year in the U.S. alone due to influenza vaccination.

(For more on GBS, see the chapter on covid vaccines and paralysis.)

54.

Guillain-Barré syndrome is 2 to 5 times more likely to occur after receiving a seasonal influenza vaccine

"According to these results the attributable risk in adults ranges from two to five Guillain-Barré syndrome cases per one million vaccinations."

Galeotti F, Massari M, et al. **Risk of Guillain-Barré syndrome after 2010-2011 influenza vaccination**. *Eur J Epidemiol* 2013 May; 28(5): 433-44.

- Guillain-Barré syndrome (GBS) is a severe ailment: up to 10% of patients die and 20% are still incapacitated after 6 months.

- In this study, Italian scientists conducted two analyses — a matched case-control and a self-controlled case series — to explore a possible link between seasonal influenza vaccination and GBS.

- In the case-control analysis, there was a significantly elevated risk of GBS within 6 weeks after influenza vaccination (odds ratio, OR = 3.8). The risk was even higher within 2 weeks of vaccination (OR = 4.7).

- When the case-control analysis was restricted to cases coming from 37 neurological centers with complete reporting as verified through hospital administrative discharge data (to avoid a possible selection bias) the association between influenza vaccination and GBS increased (OR = 4.9).

- The self-controlled case series analysis also showed a significantly elevated risk of GBS after influenza vaccination (relative risk, RR = 2.1).

- Seasonal influenza vaccines cause between 2 and 5 excess cases of GBS per million people vaccinated.

- The median onset of the first neurological symptom following influenza vaccination was 14 days, with a range of 9-39 days.

55.

Severe Guillain-Barré syndrome with prolonged disability is 8 times more likely to occur after receiving a seasonal influenza vaccine

"The incidence rate of severe Guillain-Barré syndrome following influenza vaccination was statistically increased in comparison to the adult tetanus-diphtheria vaccine control group. As an optional vaccine for high-risk patients in a rapidly enlarging population, influenza vaccination should only be given with informed consent. Patients need to understand the potential benefits, limitations, and risks involved with influenza vaccination."

Geier MR, Geier DA, Zahalsky AC. **Influenza vaccination and Guillain Barre syndrome.** *Clin Immunol* 2003 May; 107(2): 116-21.

- In this study the Vaccine Adverse Events Reporting System (VAERS) database was analyzed to determine the risk of developing Guillain-Barré syndrome (GBS) after receiving a seasonal influenza vaccine.

- Guillain-Barré syndrome is a serious autoimmune disease of the nervous system leading to muscle weakness and paralysis that can last months or years.

- There was a significantly increased risk of developing acute GBS (relative risk, RR = 4.3) and severe GBS with residual disability 1 year later (RR = 8.5) after receiving an influenza vaccine in comparison to a control group.

- The median onset of GBS following influenza vaccination was 12 days.

- There were statistically significant variations in the incidence of Guillain-Barré syndrome — and endotoxin levels varied up to 10-fold — among different influenza vaccine lots and manufacturers.

- The presence of endotoxin in influenza vaccines is a serious concern because it can stimulate antibody production to unrelated antigens. Biological plausibility for GBS after influenza vaccine may be due to the synergistic effects of endotoxin and vaccine-induced autoimmunity.

56.

Guillain-Barré syndrome is statistically more likely to occur within six weeks after receiving a seasonal influenza vaccine

"We estimate that after age, sex, and season have been controlled for, the risk of the Guillain-Barré syndrome is increased by a factor of 1.7 in the six weeks after influenza vaccination."

Lasky T, Terracciano GJ, et al. **The Guillain-Barré syndrome and the 1992-1993 and 1993-1994 influenza vaccines.** *N Engl J Med* 1998 Dec 17; 339(25): 1797-1802.

- In this study, researchers interviewed 180 adults hospitalized with Guillain-Barré syndrome (GBS). Onset within six weeks after influenza vaccination was defined as vaccine-associated and confirmed by vaccine providers.

- There was a significantly increased likelihood of developing GBS within six weeks following influenza vaccination (relative risk, RR = 2.4). After adjusting for age, sex and influenza season, the increased risk remained statistically significant (RR = 1.7).

- Onset of GBS symptoms occurred most often in the second week after influenza vaccination — all between days 9 and 12 — suggestive of a true association between vaccination and the disorder.

- This study was supported by the CDC.

57.

Dieleman J, Romio S, et al. **Guillain-Barré syndrome and adjuvanted pandemic influenza A (H1N1) 2009 vaccine: multinational case-control study in Europe.** *BMJ* 2011 Jul 12; 343: d3908.

- In this paper, pandemic influenza vaccination was not shown to increase the risk of GBS but data from the United Kingdom revealed a significantly increased risk of developing GBS after receiving a seasonal influenza vaccine (OR = 5.1 after adjustment for prior infections).

58.

Seasonal influenza vaccination significantly increases the risk of GBS

"The long onset interval and low prevalence of other preexisting illnesses are consistent with a possible causal association between Guillain-Barré syndrome and influenza vaccine."

Haber P, DeStefano F, et al. **Guillain-Barré syndrome following influenza vaccination.** *JAMA* 2004 Nov 24; 292(20): 2478-81.

• GBS can be triggered by either an acute illness or influenza vaccination.

• Two findings in this paper suggest that many VAERS reports of GBS after influenza vaccination are causally related adverse events: 1) the median onset for GBS is 13 days post-vaccination versus 1 day for non-GBS adverse events, and 2) few GBS cases after influenza vaccination also had a preceding illness.

59.

Juurlink DN, Stukel TA, et al. **Guillain-Barré syndrome after influenza vaccination in adults: a population-based study.** *Arch Intern Med* 2006 Nov 13; 166(20): 2217-21.

"Influenza vaccination is associated with a small but significantly increased risk for hospitalization because of Guillain-Barré syndrome."

• In this study, Canadian scientists found a significantly increased risk of being diagnosed with Guillain-Barré syndrome 2-7 weeks after influenza vaccination compared with a control period (relative incidence, RI = 1.45).

60.

Chen R, Kent J, Rhodes P. **Investigation of a possible association between influenza vaccination and Guillain-Barre syndrome in the United States, 1990-91.** *Post Mark Surveill* 1992 Jan; 6: 5-6.

• There was a significantly increased risk of GBS among persons 18 to 64 years of age who received a seasonal influenza vaccine (relative risk, RR = 3.5).

61.

A national swine influenza vaccination program in 1976-1977 severely disabled many people with Guillain-Barré syndrome

"Epidemiologic evidence indicated that many cases of Guillain-Barré syndrome were related to vaccination. When compared to the unvaccinated population, the vaccinated population had a significantly elevated attack rate in every adult age group."

Schonberger LB, Bregman DJ, et al. **Guillain-Barré syndrome following vaccination in the national influenza immunization program, United States, 1976-1977.** *Am J Epidemiol* 1979; 110(2): 105-123.

• Researchers found a significantly increased risk of GBS after swine influenza vaccination when compared to an unvaccinated population (RR = 7.6). This translates to about 10 excess cases of GBS per million people vaccinated.

62.

Langmuir AD, Bregman DJ, et al. **An epidemiologic and clinical evaluation of Guillain-Barré syndrome reported in association with the administration of swine influenza vaccines.** *Am J Epidemiol* 1984 Jun; 119(6): 841-79.

"Vaccinated cases with 'extensive' paresis or paralysis occurred in a characteristic epidemiologic pattern closely approximated by a lognormal curve, suggesting a causal relationship between the disease and the vaccine."

• In this study, researchers analyzed approximately 1,300 suspected cases of Guillain-Barré syndrome following the 1976-1977 national swine influenza vaccination program.

• There was a significantly increased probability of extensive disability over a 6-week period following swine influenza vaccination. Relative risk ranged from 3.96 to 7.75 depending on different estimates of normal background incidence.

63.

Many people vaccinated against swine influenza in 1976-1977 were stricken with Guillain-Barré syndrome

"These findings suggest that there was an increased risk of developing Guillain-Barré syndrome during the 6 weeks following vaccination in adults."

Safranek TJ, Lawrence DN, et al. **Reassessment of the association between Guillain-Barré syndrome and receipt of swine influenza vaccine in 1976-1977: results of a two-state study. Expert Neurology Group.** *Am J Epidemiol* 1991 May 1; 133(9): 940-51.

- For every million people vaccinated against swine influenza, there were between 8.6 and 9.7 excess cases of Guillain-Barré syndrome within 6 weeks attributed to the vaccine.

64.

Marks JS, Halpin TJ. **Guillain-Barré syndrome in recipients of A/New Jersey influenza vaccine.** *JAMA* 1980 Jun 27; 243(24): 2490-94.

"An elevated risk of Guillain-Barré syndrome remained in vaccinees regardless of manufacturer or vaccine type."

- In this study, researchers found a significantly increased risk of Guillain-Barré syndrome after swine influenza vaccination (13.3 cases per million) when compared to an unvaccinated population (2.6 cases per million).

65.

Breman JG, Hayner NS. **Guillain-Barré syndrome and its relationship to swine influenza vaccination in Michigan, 1976-1977.** *Am J Epidemiol* 1984 Jun; 119(6): 880-89.

- In this study, for every million people vaccinated against swine influenza there were 11.7 excess cases of Guillain-Barré syndrome within 6 weeks.

66.

A global swine influenza vaccination program in 2009-2010 severely disabled many people with Guillain-Barré syndrome

"The significance and consistency of our findings support a conclusion of an association between 2009 H1N1 vaccination and Guillain Barré syndrome."

Dodd CN, Romio SA, et al. **International collaboration to assess the risk of Guillain Barré syndrome following Influenza A (H1N1) 2009 monovalent vaccines.** *Vaccine* 2013 Sep 13; 31(40): 4448-58.

• Researchers found a significantly elevated risk of GBS within 6 weeks following swine influenza (H1N1) vaccination in both a pooled data analysis (relative incidence, RI = 2.42) and meta-analysis (RI = 2.42).

67.

Wise ME, Viray M, et al. **Guillain-Barre syndrome during the 2009-2010 H1N1 influenza vaccination campaign: population-based surveillance among 45 million Americans.** *Am J Epidemiol* 2012 Jun 1; 175(11): 1110-19.

• CDC scientists analyzed cases of GBS following a national H1N1 influenza vaccination campaign and found a significantly elevated risk within 6 weeks following the shot compared with a later control period (rate ratio, RR = 1.57). The risk was even higher within 4 weeks of vaccination (RR = 1.83).

• Preceding cases of respiratory illness were significantly less common among people who developed GBS within 6 weeks after H1N1 vaccination than among those who did not (38% vs 67%), providing additional evidence of a causal link between H1N1 vaccination and GBS.

• Fifteen percent of GBS cases required mechanical ventilation (to help patients breathe), and 3% died.

68.

Many people vaccinated against swine influenza in 2009-2010 were stricken with Guillain-Barré syndrome

"In Quebec, the 2009 influenza A (H1N1) vaccine was associated with a small but significant risk of Guillain Barré syndrome."

De Wals P, Deceuninck G, et al. **Risk of Guillain-Barré syndrome following H1N1 influenza vaccination in Quebec.** *JAMA* 2012 Jul 11; 308(2): 175-81.

- Canadian researchers found a significantly elevated risk of Guillain Barré syndrome within 4 weeks following pandemic swine influenza (H1N1) vaccination (RR = 2.75). The risk was even higher using the self-controlled case-series method for all confirmed cases (RR = 3.02).

- The approximate number of Guillain Barré syndrome cases attributable to pandemic influenza vaccination was 2 per million people vaccinated.

69.

Polakowski LL, Sandhu SK, et al. **Chart-confirmed Guillain-Barre syndrome after 2009 H1N1 influenza vaccination among the Medicare population, 2009-2010.** *Am J Epidemiol* 2013 Sep 15; 178(6): 962-73.

- In this study, researchers analyzed a population of Medicare recipients who were hospitalized with GBS after receiving an H1N1 influenza vaccination and found a significantly elevated risk within 6 weeks following the shot compared with a later control period (incidence rate ratio, IRR = 2.41).

70.

Meta-analyses found a significantly increased risk of Guillain-Barré syndrome after swine influenza vaccination, 2009-2010

"The results of the present meta-analysis point to a small but statistically significant association between influenza vaccines, particularly the pandemic ones, and Guillain-Barré syndrome, which is consistent with current explanations upon possible mechanisms for this condition to appear."

Martín Arias LH, Sanz R, et al. **Guillain-Barré syndrome and influenza vaccines: a meta-analysis.** *Vaccine* 2015 Jul 17; 33(31): 3773-78.

- Researchers conducted a meta-analysis and concluded that the risk of Guillain-Barré syndrome was significantly elevated after receiving either a pandemic influenza vaccine (RR = 1.84) or seasonal influenza vaccine (RR = 1.22).

71.

Salmon DA, Proschan M, et al. **Association between Guillain-Barré syndrome and influenza A (H1N1) 2009 monovalent inactivated vaccines in the USA: a meta-analysis.** *Lancet* 2013 Apr 27; 381(9876): 1461-68.

- Guillain-Barré syndrome is a serious health condition in which a person's own immune system damages their nerve cells, causing muscle weakness, paralysis, and sometimes death.

- Researchers conducted a meta-analysis and determined that inactivated pandemic influenza (H1N1) vaccines significantly increased the risk of developing Guillain-Barré syndrome (incidence rate ratio, IRR = 2.35) This translates to about 1.6 excess cases of GBS per million people vaccinated.

72.

Vaccination against swine influenza in 2009-2010 quadrupled the risk of Guillain-Barré syndrome

"The results indicate an increased risk of Guillain-Barré syndrome/ Fisher syndrome in temporal association with pandemic influenza A (H1N1) vaccination in Germany."

Prestel J, Volkers P, et al. **Risk of Guillain-Barré syndrome following pandemic influenza A(H1N1) 2009 vaccination in Germany.** *Pharmacoepidemiol Drug Saf* 2014 Nov; 23(11): 1192-1204.

- German researchers analyzed cases of Guillain-Barré syndrome (and its variant Fisher syndrome) following a 2009 national pandemic influenza (H1N1) vaccination campaign and found a significantly elevated risk 5-42 days post-vaccination compared with a later control period (RI = 4.65).

- The results remained highly significant when adjusted for various factors such as the exclusion of concurrent seasonal influenza vaccination (RI = 4.83).

73.

Greene SK, Rett M, et al. **Risk of confirmed Guillain-Barre syndrome following receipt of monovalent inactivated influenza A (H1N1) and seasonal influenza vaccines in the Vaccine Safety Datalink Project, 2009-2010.** *Am J Epidemiol* 2012 Jun 1; 175(11): 1100-9.

- In this study, researchers utilized the CDC's Vaccine Safety Datalink database (containing health data on millions of people) to assess the risk of developing Guillain-Barré syndrome following receipt of pandemic influenza (H1N1) and seasonal influenza vaccines during the 2009-2010 influenza season.

- In a self-controlled risk interval analysis, researchers found a significantly elevated risk of GBS within 1-42 days following receipt of pandemic influenza (H1N1) vaccine compared with a later control period (RR = 4.7). This translates to about 4 excess cases of GBS per million people vaccinated.

74.

Pandemic (swine) influenza vaccination in 2009-2010 significantly increased cases of Guillain-Barré syndrome

"Pandemic influenza (H1N1) vaccination increased the Guillain-Barré syndrome rate."

Kim C, Rhie S, et al. **Pandemic influenza A vaccination and incidence of Guillain-Barré syndrome in Korea.** *Vaccine* 2015 Apr 8; 33(15): 1815-23.

- Korean researchers determined that the rate of GBS was significantly higher in persons 20-34 years of age after receiving a pandemic influenza (H1N1) vaccine compared to a reference period (rate ratio, RR = 1.46).

- This study was conducted in collaboration with the Korea Centers for Disease Control and Prevention.

75.

Tokars JI, Lewis P, et al. **The risk of Guillain-Barré syndrome associated with influenza A (H1N1) 2009 monovalent vaccine and 2009-2010 seasonal influenza vaccines: results from self-controlled analyses.** *Pharmacoepidemiol Drug Saf* 2012 May; 21(5): 546-52.

- Researchers found a significantly elevated risk of developing GBS 1-6 weeks following receipt of a pandemic influenza (H1N1) vaccine compared with a later control period 7-12 weeks post-vaccination (RR = 3.0). This translates to about 2.8 excess cases of GBS per million people vaccinated.

- This study was conducted by the CDC.

Doctors and Nurses Infect Patients

Doctors, nurses, and other healthcare workers often work while sick with contagious respiratory infections, such as influenza, despite putting their patients at risk. For example, in an anonymous survey (Szymczak) of 538 healthcare specialists at The Children's Hospital of Philadelphia, 95% of the respondents recognized that working while sick puts patients at risk, yet 83% admitted they went to work sick within the past year. Other studies have shown that more than 80% of doctors go to work when they are experiencing influenza-like illness.

Some studies show that vaccinated healthcare workers are significantly more likely than unvaccinated workers to go to work sick with a potentially contagious influenza-like illness. Chiu conducted an anonymous survey of 1,914 healthcare personnel and found that more than 44% who went to work with influenza-like illness were vaccinated against influenza, compared with 29% who were not vaccinated ($p = .03$). Physicians had the highest frequency of working while sick.

LaVela conducted an anonymous survey of 753 healthcare workers who care for patients at high-risk for respiratory complications. They found that 86% of medical staff who experienced symptoms of a respiratory infection attended work, and 52% worked at least three days while symptomatic. There were no significant differences between healthcare workers who were vaccinated against influenza and those who were unvaccinated regarding whether they had a respiratory infection.

Reasons for working sick are varied. In Chiu's survey, respondents claimed: "I wasn't feeling bad enough to miss work," and "I didn't think I was contagious or could make other people sick." Yet, 57% of all sick healthcare personnel visited a medical provider for relief of symptoms, and 25% were told they had influenza. Healthcare practitioners may also work while sick out of concern for colleagues, not wanting to be perceived as weak, and "a strong cultural norm to come to work unless remarkably ill."

Health authorities and medical centers promote influenza vaccines to reduce the spread of influenza yet there is an institutional expectation for doctors, nurses, and other healthcare personnel to show up at work when sick, even when exhibiting symptoms of influenza-like illness. Although this choice puts co-workers and patients at higher risk of contracting a respiratory infection — and increases the likelihood of medical errors — it appears to be unofficially sanctioned. Sincere, non-hypocritical guidelines must be established to prevent sick doctors and nurses from acting as vectors of disease during outbreaks of respiratory illness.

76.

Doctors and nurses often work while sick with contagious respiratory symptoms despite putting their patients at risk

"Attending physicians and advanced practice clinicians frequently work while sick despite recognizing that this choice puts patients at risk."

Szymczak JE, Smathers S, et al. **Reasons why physicians and advanced practice clinicians work while sick: a mixed-methods analysis.** *JAMA Pediatr* 2015 Sep; 169(9): 815-821.

- When healthcare practitioners go to work sick they can spread disease to patients and colleagues. The medical literature contains numerous reports of outbreaks such as influenza within healthcare facilities that were traced to sick healthcare workers as the ultimate source of transmission.

- Researchers conducted a survey of 538 doctors, nurses, and other healthcare specialists at The Children's Hospital of Philadelphia to investigate the frequency with which and reasons why they work while ill.

- Although 95% of the respondents recognized that working while sick puts patients at risk, 83% admitted they went to work sick within the past year.

- Nearly 1 in 10 reported having worked sick at least six times in the past year.

- More than 55% would work while sick with significant respiratory symptoms.

- A "strong cultural norm to come to work unless remarkably ill" and "ambiguity about what constitutes too sick to work" were listed as common reasons why healthcare practitioners work with possibly contagious symptoms despite recognizing that this choice puts patients at risk.

77.

Vaccinated healthcare personnel are much more likely than unvaccinated personnel to go to work sick with a potentially contagious influenza-like illness

"Receiving influenza vaccination at any time during the influenza season was associated with working with influenza-like illness."

Chiu S, Black CL, et al. **Working with influenza-like illness: presenteeism among US health care personnel during the 2014-2015 influenza season.** *Am J Infect Control* 2017 Nov 1; 45(11): 1254-58.

- Influenza can be transmitted to coworkers and patients at healthcare sites, so researchers conducted an anonymous survey of 1,914 healthcare personnel to determine their frequency of working while experiencing influenza-like illness (ILI), and reasons why they work while ill.

- More than 40% of healthcare workers go to work when sick with ILI (for a median of 3 days). Pharmacists (67%) and physicians (63%) had the highest frequency of working while sick.

- More than 44% of healthcare personnel who work in an obstetrics unit or around seriously ill patients work while sick.

- Reasons for working sick included: "I wasn't feeling bad enough to miss work," and "I didn't think I was contagious or could make other people sick." Yet, 57% of all sick healthcare personnel visited a medical provider for relief of symptoms, and 25% were told they had influenza.

- More than 44% of healthcare personnel who went to work with influenza-like illness were vaccinated against influenza, compared with 29% who were not vaccinated ($p = .03$).

- Although the CDC recommends that healthcare personnel with ILI not work until they are afebrile for 24 hours (past the contagious stage), healthcare workers often disregard this advice and continue to work with ILI.

78.

Doctors go to work sick
with flu-like symptoms

"The act of working while ill has important implications for healthcare personnel, whose repeated interactions with patients make productivity declines from illness more dangerous and disease transmission more likely."

Jena AB, Meltzer DO, et al. **Why physicians work when sick.** *Arch Intern Med* 2012 Jul 23; 172(14): 1107-08. [Research letter.]

- Researchers conducted an anonymous survey of 150 resident physicians to determine their frequency of working with flu-like symptoms.

- Fifty-one percent of the doctors reported working with flu-like symptoms at least once in the past year; 16% worked sick at least 3 times.

- The most common reasons for working when ill were an obligation to colleagues and to patient care. Female doctors were more likely to work when ill because they did not want to be perceived as weak.

79.

Jena AB, Baldwin DC Jr, et al. **Presenteeism among resident physicians.** *JAMA* 2010 Sep 15; 304(11): 1166-68. [Research letter.]

"Despite recent CDC guidelines urging healthcare personnel with flu-like illness to avoid working, presenteeism (working while sick) is prevalent among healthcare workers."

- Researchers conducted an anonymous survey of 537 resident physicians to determine their frequency of working while sick.

- Fifty-eight percent of the doctors reported working while sick at least once in the past year; 31% worked sick more than once in the previous year.

- Doctors may work sick for several reasons, including misplaced dedication, and fear of letting down teammates.

80.

Doctors and other healthcare workers attend work with respiratory infections despite knowing the risk to patients

"It is alarming that 86% of healthcare workers attended work while symptomatic, given the consequences that respiratory infection can have on persons [at high risk for respiratory complications]."

LaVela S, Goldstein B, et al. **Working with symptoms of a respiratory infection: staff who care for high-risk individuals.** *Am J Infect Control* 2007 Sep; 35(7): 448-454.

- Researchers conducted an anonymous survey of 753 healthcare workers. Overall, 36% of healthcare workers had symptoms of a respiratory infection during a single influenza season. Of those, 86% attended work; 52% worked for 3 or more days while symptomatic.

81.

Gudgeon P, Wells DA, et al. **Do you come to work with a respiratory tract infection?** *Occup Environ Med* 2009 Jun; 66(6): 424. [Letter.]

"In susceptible populations [respiratory illnesses] are associated with significant morbidity. Additionally, there is a risk of impaired judgment, decreased level of functioning and reduced productivity when working while ill."

- Researchers surveyed physicians and medical students to determine their frequency of working with a respiratory tract infection.

- They reported a high incidence of working while ill despite knowing that working with a respiratory tract infection posed a risk to others.

- Reasons given for working while sick included concern about their patients and how they would be perceived by others if they missed work.

- Institutional mechanisms need to be developed to prevent sick doctors from acting as vectors of disease during outbreaks of respiratory illness.

82.

Doctors often go to work with contagious diseases such as influenza

"A large number of physicians are working whilst suffering from diseases that can be harmful to their patients."

Rosvold EO, Bjertness E. **Physicians who do not take sick leave: hazardous heroes?** *Scand J Public Health* 2001 Mar; 29(1): 71-75.

- Researchers conducted an anonymous survey of 1,015 physicians to determine their frequency of working while sick and the diseases that they bring to work.

- During the previous year, 80% of physicians worked during an illness for which they would have sick-listed their patients.

- Infectious diseases, including influenza and other respiratory tract infections, comprised 66% of the reported illnesses brought to work by sick doctors. Since most infections are contagious, these physicians are risking the health of their patients and staff members.

- Doctors also reported going to work with headache, pain, and depression, and vomiting while at work, which could affect their ability to assist patients.

83.

Bracewell LM, Campbell DI, et al. **Sickness presenteeism in a New Zealand hospital.** *N Z Med J* 2010 May 14; 123(1314): 31-42.

"This study provides evidence that sickness presenteeism (working while sick) is prevalent in the District Health Board and is similar to findings elsewhere."

- In this study of 400 healthcare workers, doctors were more likely to work while sick than any other occupational group.

84.

Healthcare workers work when sick, shed respiratory viruses, and risk spreading influenza-like-illness to their patients

"In this cohort, healthcare workers working while ill was common, as was viral shedding among those with symptoms."

Esbenshade JC, Edwards KM, et al. **Respiratory virus shedding in a cohort of on-duty healthcare workers undergoing prospective surveillance.** *Infect Control Hosp Epidemiol* 2013 Apr; 34(4): 373-78.

- Healthcare workers are known to work while sick, potentially spreading contagious pathogens to vulnerable patients. Transmission of respiratory viruses by healthcare workers is a safety concern.

- In this study, scientists collected nasal specimens from 159 healthcare workers in a children's hospital to assess viral shedding of respiratory pathogens.

- Forty-six percent of all healthcare workers reported working while sick with an influenza-like illness during the previous influenza season; 80% of doctors worked while sick.

- Viral shedding was most common among younger healthcare workers.

- Findings in this paper indicate that healthcare workers with detected viral pathogens work while sick, and these people may spread influenza-like illness to their patients.

85.

Gustafsson Sendén M, Løvseth LT, et al. **What makes physicians go to work while sick: a comparative study of sickness presenteeism in four European countries (HOUPE).** *Swiss Med Wkly* 2013 Aug 22; 143: w13840.

- In Italy, 86% of physicians acknowledged that they "sometimes or often went to work while ill." In Norway, Iceland, and Sweden, the figures were 76%, 75%, and 70%, respectively.

86.

Healthcare workers often go to work sick with a potentially contagious influenza-like illness

"Only 31% of healthcare workers reported routinely taking sick leave for influenza-like illness."

Turnberg W, Daniell W, Duchin J. **Influenza vaccination and sick leave practices and perceptions reported by health care workers in ambulatory care settings.** *Am J Infect Control* 2010 Aug; 38(6): 486-88.

- Researchers examined influenza vaccination and sick leave practices among 627 healthcare workers from 5 medical centers.

- Although 67% of healthcare workers reported receiving an annual influenza vaccine, 69% go to work when sick with an influenza-like illness, placing their co-workers and patients at risk for infection.

- Healthcare workers who are sick with symptoms of a contagious respiratory illness should follow the principle of 'first do no harm' by avoiding contact with their patients.

87.

Widera E, Chang A, Chen HL. **Presenteeism: a public health hazard.** *J Gen Intern Med* 2010 Nov; 25(11): 1244-47.

"Healthcare workers as a group are very likely to continue to work when infected with diseases such as influenza...despite the serious public health risks."

- Presenteeism occurs when an employee goes to work sick. This paper reviewed the literature indicating that healthcare workers frequently go to work sick with infectious illnesses such as influenza that can be transmitted to vulnerable patients.

SARS, MERS, and
Gain-of-Function Research

The studies in this chapter discuss severe acute respiratory syndrome (SARS) and Middle East respiratory syndrome (MERS), two coronaviruses that existed before covid-19. Scientists were unable to develop safe and effective vaccines against these diseases. This chapter also discusses gain-of-function research, experimentation designed to enhance the transmissibility and virulence of a pathogen. U.S. and Chinese scientists collaborated on the creation of a hybrid coronavirus. Gain-of-function research can improve our understanding of disease-causing agents or cause deadly pandemics.

88.

Scientists were unable to develop a safe coronavirus vaccine against SARS

"In each of the experiments conducted here, immunization with the whole inactivated SARS vaccine induced increased inflammatory infiltrates and pulmonary eosinophilia upon subsequent challenge, demonstrating the potential for dangerous clinical complications."

Bolles M, Deming D, et al. **A double-inactivated severe acute respiratory syndrome coronavirus vaccine provides incomplete protection in mice and induces increased eosinophilic proinflammatory pulmonary response upon challenge.** *J Virol* 2011 Dec; 85(23): 12201-15.

- In 2002, a new disease — severe acute respiratory syndrome (SARS) — emerged in China. The mortality rate exceeded 50% in elderly populations. The etiological agent was a novel coronavirus presumed to originate in bats prior to the human epidemic.

- This paper describes several experiments that were conducted on mice to determine whether an effective and safe vaccine against SARS could be developed for humans.

- Elderly mice that received a non-adjuvanted SARS vaccine were unable to produce detectable antibodies against the disease.

- In elderly mice, SARS vaccines with or without an aluminum adjuvant failed to induce protective immunity against heterologous or homologous viral challenges. In addition, when compared to the control group, both vaccine formulations significantly amplified pulmonary immune pathology.

- The SARS vaccine failed to protect against viral replication, morbidity and mortality. It also caused increases in cytokines IL-5 and IL-13 while enhancing inflammatory damage within the lungs.

- Findings in this study raise the possibility that SARS-vaccinated populations may develop eosinophilic immunopathology when exposed to non-epidemic coronavirus strains.

89.

A potential coronavirus vaccine against SARS caused pulmonary pathology upon exposure to the virus

"Not only did nucleocapsid (N) vaccination fail to control SARS coronavirus replication within the lungs, but N vaccination also resulted in an enhanced immunopathology in the lungs of the senescent animals upon viral challenge."

Deming D, Sheahan T, et al. **Vaccine efficacy in senescent mice challenged with recombinant SARS-CoV bearing epidemic and zoonotic spike variants.** *PLoS Med* 2006 Dec; 3(12): e525.

- In 2002, a novel coronavirus — severe acute respiratory syndrome (SARS) — emerged in China. This new disease, characterized by severe pneumonia and a high fatality rate, quickly spread to other nations.

- This paper describes a SARS vaccine that was tested on mice to determine whether immunity could be achieved in both young and elderly populations. The vaccine was tested against the current coronavirus strain causing the epidemic and heterologous strains that might yet emerge from animals.

- Scientists developed vaccines utilizing the S (spike) and N (nucleocapsid) proteins associated with SARS. The S vaccine provided poor immunity in elderly animals. The N vaccine protected neither young nor elderly mice and caused immunopathology in their lungs when challenged by the virus.

- Several concerns complicate the creation of a coronavirus vaccine, including the potential for reversion or recombination of attenuated vaccine strains, induction of immunopathology, lack of cross-protection against variant strains, poor efficacy in elderly populations, and waning immunity in all age groups.

- Vaccines that contain the nucleocapsid protein should be used with caution in human populations.

- This study identified challenges in designing a safe and effective vaccine for future coronaviruses, especially in vulnerable elderly populations.

90.

Scientists were unable to develop a safe coronavirus vaccine against MERS

"Inactivated MERS vaccine appears to carry a hypersensitive-type lung pathology risk from MERS infection that is similar to that found with inactivated SARS vaccines from SARS infection."

Agrawal AS, Tao X, et al. **Immunization with inactivated Middle East Respiratory Syndrome coronavirus vaccine leads to lung immuno-pathology on challenge with live virus.** *Hum Vaccin Immunother* 2016 Sep; 12(9): 2351-56.

- In 2002, a new coronavirus, Severe Acute Respiratory Syndrome (SARS), began circulating in human populations. Scientists were unable to develop a safe vaccine against SARS because vaccinated mice would develop lung pathology after being exposed to the virus.

- In 2012, another novel coronavirus, Middle East Respiratory Syndrome (MERS), emerged in humans. Although clinical trials of SARS vaccines were suspended, scientists now wondered whether a safe and effective MERS vaccine could be developed.

- This current study was conducted to determine whether a safe vaccine against MERS could be developed, one that would not cause lung pathology following exposure to the virus (similar to what occurred with SARS vaccines).

- Scientists vaccinated mice against MERS, which induced neutralizing antibodies against infection. However, when the mice were exposed to the MERS coronavirus there were significant increases in cytokines IL-5 and IL-13 plus increased lung pathology with eosinophil (white blood cell) infiltrations.

- Previous studies have shown that increases of IL-5 and IL-13 are associated with hypersensitivity reactions that include eosinophil infiltrations.

- This study provides evidence that an inactivated MERS vaccine to prevent MERS in humans is likely to cause lung immunopathology when vaccinated individuals are subsequently exposed to the wild MERS coronavirus.

91.

U.S. and Chinese scientists collaborated on the creation of a hybrid coronavirus

"On the basis of these findings, scientific review panels may deem similar studies building chimeric viruses based on circulating strains too risky to pursue, as increased pathogenicity in mammalian models cannot be excluded. The potential to prepare for and mitigate future outbreaks must be weighed against the risk of creating more dangerous pathogens."

Menachery VD, Yount BL Jr, et al. **A SARS-like cluster of circulating bat coronaviruses shows potential for human emergence.** *Nat Med* 2015 Dec; 21(12): 1508-13.

- Scientists have discovered a cluster of SARS-like coronaviruses circulating in Chinese bats. To examine their potential to cross species and infect humans, they genetically created a hybrid virus from Chinese horseshoe bats expressed in a mouse-adapted SARS coronavirus backbone.

- The creation of a hybrid coronavirus enabled scientists to assess the ability of the novel spike protein to infect humans independently of other adaptive mutations and exhibited robust viral replication both in vitro and in vivo.

- Aged mice vaccinated against infection with the hybrid coronavirus were not protected and immune pathology was augmented.

- This work was undertaken due to a potential risk of a SARS coronavirus re-emergence from viruses circulating in bat populations. However, gain-of-function research to prepare against future emerging viruses can increase the risk of creating more contagious and virulent pathogens.

- Research conducted in this paper was supported by the National Institutes of Health, the National Institute of Allergy & Infectious Disease (Anthony S. Fauci, Director), EcoHealth Alliance, and the National Natural Science Foundation of China.

- Hybrid SARS-like coronaviruses were cultured on Vero E6 cells obtained from the U.S. Army Medical Research Institute of Infectious Diseases.

92.

Gain-of-function research can improve our understanding of disease-causing agents or cause deadly pandemics

"Biosecurity risks associated with dual-use life science research are especially difficult (if not impossible) to estimate with confidence. Using biosafety level 3 (BSL-3) lab infection data, Lipsitch and Inglesby estimated a probability of between 0.01 % and 0.1 % per laboratory year of creating a pandemic which would cause between 2 million and 1.4 billion fatalities."

Selgelid MJ. **Gain-of-Function Research: Ethical Analysis.** *Sci Eng Ethics* 2016 Aug; 22(4): 923-964.

- Gain-of-function (GOF) research involves experimentation designed to increase the transmissibility and/or virulence of pathogens, usually with the intention to better understand disease-causing agents, their effect on humans, and their potential to cause pandemics.

- In 2014, following several biosafety accidents in government labs, U.S. President Barack Obama temporarily suspended funding on GOF research involving SARS, MERS, and influenza viruses.

- This Ethical Analysis White Paper was commissioned by the National Institutes of Health to review the literature on GOF research and develop an ethical framework for assessing the risks/benefits of all GOF projects.

- Potential benefits of GOF research include gain of scientific knowledge, public health surveillance, and creation of medical preventatives/therapies. Risks include pandemics and extensive economic losses due to an accidental or intentional pathogen release, terrorism, and loss of public trust in science.

- The ethical framework proposed in this paper is designed to indicate where any GOF study would fall on an ethical spectrum. Yet, clear answers may not always be possible regarding whether a GOF project should proceed.

- The potential consequences of scientifically enhancing the virulence and contagiousness of deadly pathogens must be considered in all GOF research.

Covid Vaccine Effectiveness and Treatment

The studies in this chapter provide evidence of no long-term covid vaccine effectiveness. For example, Nordström evaluated a population of more that 1.6 million vaccinated and unvaccinated individuals and found no clear benefit in adults 50 to 79 years of age by the fifth month post vaccination. Ferdinands found that in the 18 to 44 year age group, by four, six, and eight months after a third vaccine dose, effectiveness against hospital admissions was 33%, -24%, and -68%, respectively. As time progressed, negative efficacy increased and this cohort was more likely than controls to contract covid and be hospitalized.

Rancourt found that covid vaccines increased all-cause mortality. d'Almeida found that vaccine passports needed for travel are associated with an increase in all-cause mortality because covid vaccines do not prevent transmission and provide a false sense of security. Kustin found that people who are fully vaccinated against the original covid strain are significantly more likely than unvaccinated people to contract an alternate strain. And Rick's paper found that a previous covid infection provides a 92% decreased risk of contracting another covid infection compared to people who had no prior covid infection.

Kerr found that the regular use of ivermectin as a treatment for covid decreased hospitalization by 100% and mortality by 92% when compared to non-users. Bryant found that ivermectin treatment reduced the risk of death by an average of 62%, compared to non-users. And Uusküla found that natural immunity offers stronger and longer-lasting protection against covid infections, symptoms, and hospitalizations than vaccine-induced immunity.

93.

Two doses of a covid vaccine provide little protection after a few months

"We found progressively waning vaccine effectiveness against SARS-CoV-2 [covid] infection of any severity across all subgroups, but the rate of waning differed according to vaccine type."

Nordström P, Ballin M, Nordström A. **Risk of infection, hospitalisation, and death up to 9 months after a second dose of COVID-19 vaccine: a retrospective, total population cohort study in Sweden.** *Lancet* 2022 Feb 26; 399(10327): 814-823.

- This study investigated the effectiveness of covid vaccination during the first 9 months after vaccination. Three covid vaccines were evaluated. The study population consisted of 1,685,948 vaccinated and unvaccinated individuals.

- The authors found a substantial and progressive waning of vaccine protection against covid infection of any severity across all groups of people, with variations in the rate of decline related to the type of vaccine administered.

- Vaccine effectiveness was undetectable with AstraZeneca vaccination after more than 4 months and Pfizer vaccination after 6 months.

- Generally, vaccine effectiveness was lower in older people than in younger people. By the fifth month post vaccination, the covid vaccine showed no clear benefit in adults 50-79 years of age (Table 3).

- After six months post vaccination, covid-vaccinated people 80 years of age and older were found to be 80% more likely than unvaccinated people to contract covid (Table 3).

- Vaccine effectiveness was also lower in men than in women. There was no detectable vaccine protection in men after 6 months.

94.

Vaccine effectiveness declines within months against covid-related hospitalizations and emergency care

"Protection conferred by mRNA vaccines against moderate (emergency department or urgent care) and severe (hospital admission) covid-19 waned during the months after primary vaccination, increased substantially after the third dose, and waned again by four to five months."

Ferdinands JM, Rao S, et al. **Waning of vaccine effectiveness against moderate and severe covid-19 among adults in the US from the VISION network: test negative, case-control study.** *BMJ* 2022 Oct 3; 379: e072141.

- This study estimated the effectiveness of mRNA vaccines against moderate and severe covid by time (since second, third, or fourth doses) and age.

- More than 890,000 adults that were admitted to a hospital with covid (cases) were compared to controls (people with covid-like illness who tested negative for covid). Adults admitted to an emergency department (ED) or urgent care (UC) with covid were also compared to controls.

- During the period when the omicron variant predominated, by eight months following a third vaccine dose, effectiveness in all age groups against hospital admissions was 31% and against ED/UC visits just 17%.

- In the 18-44 year age group, by four, six, and eight months after a third vaccine dose, effectiveness against hospital admissions was 33%, -24%, and -68%, respectively. As time progressed, negative efficacy increased and this cohort was more likely than controls to contract covid and be hospitalized.

- Vaccine effectiveness was negative or very low among patients whose first medical contact was less than 14 days after the first dose.

- Pfizer's covid vaccine provided lower vaccine effectiveness than Moderna's vaccine. Both vaccines provided lower protection among adults who were immunocompromised.

95.

Covid vaccine effectiveness declines from 83% to 22% within 5 months

"In this systematic review and meta-analysis of 18 peer-reviewed studies, which included nearly 7 million individuals, we found evidence of waning immunity against SARS-CoV-2 infection from a high of 83% at one month to 22% at five months or longer after being fully vaccinated."

Ssentongo P, Ssentongo AE, et al. **SARS.CoV.2 vaccine effectiveness against infection, symptomatic and severe COVID.19: a systematic review and meta-analysis.** *BMC Infect Dis* 2022 May 7; 22(1): 439.

• The objective of this meta-analysis was to evaluate the duration of covid vaccine effectiveness against covid infection and severe covid disease. Vaccines by Pfizer, Moderna, and Janssen were considered. Eighteen studies representing 6.8 million people were reviewed.

• Vaccine effectiveness against covid infection declined rapidly after 100 days following full vaccination.

• The mean vaccine effectiveness against covid infection was 83% at one month following completion of the original vaccination series, and 22% by five months post-vaccination.

• Vaccine effectiveness declined more rapidly in seniors 65 years and older compared to younger ages, beginning approximately 25 days after vaccination.

• Vaccine effectiveness against covid infections and symptomatic covid fell below the WHO's minimal criteria of 50%.

• This study was conducted before the Omicron variant emerged, which is associated with lower vaccine effectiveness than the Delta variant.

• Boosters are likely to provide short-term increases in vaccine effectiveness, perhaps for just a few weeks after vaccination.

96.

Covid vaccine protection against infection rapidly declines after a few months

"Pfizer-induced protection against SARS-CoV-2 infection appeared to wane rapidly following its peak after the second dose. These findings suggest that a large proportion of the vaccinated population could lose its protection against infection in the coming months, perhaps increasing the potential for new epidemic waves."

Chemaitelly H, Tang P, et al. **Waning of BNT162b2 vaccine protection against SARS-CoV-2 infection in Qatar.** *N Engl J Med* 2021 Dec 9: 385(24): e83.

- This study estimated Pfizer's covid vaccine effectiveness against covid. Vaccine effectiveness against infection peaked at 77.5% in the first month after the second dose but declined to 22.5% by the fifth month, even lower after adjusting for (filtering out) people who had a prior covid infection.

- There was negative effectiveness in the first two weeks after the first dose, ranging from -4.9% to -21%, depending on the sensitivity analysis. (Vaccinated people were more likely to contract covid than the unvaccinated.)

- In some sensitivity analyses, there was substantial negative effectiveness by the 5th, 6th, and 7th months post-vaccination, as low as -83.2%.

97.

Chin ET, Leidner D, et al. **Effectiveness of the mRNA-1273 vaccine during a SARS-CoV-2 delta outbreak in a prison.** *N Engl J Med* 2021 Dec 9; 385(24): 2300-01. [Correspondence.]

- The effectiveness of the mRNA Moderna covid vaccine among male prisoners was assessed during a covid outbreak dominated by the delta variant: 468 fully vaccinated prisoners were compared to 359 unvaccinated controls.

- The vaccine was 80.5% effective in the vaccinated prisoners who previously contracted covid at least 90 days prior to the study start date, but was just 49.5% effective in the vaccinated group that had no prior covid infection.

98.

Covid vaccines and vaccine passports are associated with increased all-cause mortality

"This study of 17 countries on four continents, using all the main COVID-19 vaccine types and manufacturers, should induce governments to immediately end the baseless public health policy of prioritizing elderly residents for injection with COVID-19 vaccines."

Rancourt DG, Baudin M, et al. **COVID-19 vaccine-associated mortality in the Southern Hemisphere.** *Correlation Research in the Public Interest* 2023 Sept 17. Available: https://correlation-canada.org/covid-19-vaccine-associated-mortality-in-the-Southern-Hemisphere

- Seventeen Southern Hemisphere nations, which comprise 10.3% of covid injections, were found to have higher rates of all-cause mortality shortly after population-wide introduction of covid vaccine booster doses.

- The risk of death per vaccine dose doubles approximately every four years starting at 60 years of age. The authors estimate that covid vaccines are responsible for 17 million deaths worldwide, as of September 2, 2023.

99.

d'Almeida S. **Impact of vaccine and immunity passports in the context of COVID-19: a time series analysis in overseas France.** *Vaccines (Basel)* 2022 May 26; 10(6): 852.

"COVID-19 mortality in overseas France turned into the highest pandemic records since the adoption of immunity passports."

- In this study, time correlations were assessed between air traffic into French territories (overseas France) and covid transmission and mortality rates, before and after covid vaccine passports were implemented.

- After covid immunity passports were issued, air traffic increased 16 days before covid cases increased ($r = 0.61$) and 26 days before deaths increased ($r = 0.31$) in Martinique. Covid immunity passports cannot be trusted.

100.

Covid infection and mortality rates are worse in covid-vaccinated versus unvaccinated groups

"The COVID-bivalent vaccinated group showed a higher infection rate than the unvaccinated group in the statewide category and the age greater than or equal to 50 years category."

Ko L, Malet G, et al. **COVID-19 infection rates in vaccinated and unvaccinated inmates: a retrospective cohort study.** *Cureus* 2023 Sept 4; 15(9): e44684.

- Scientists compared covid infection rates in 96,201 covid-vaccinated versus unvaccinated inmates in California state prisons from January to July 2023.

- Infection rates in the covid-bivalent vaccinated and entirely unvaccinated groups were 3.24% and 2.72%, respectively. For individuals aged 50 and above, the infection rates were 4.07% and 3.1%, respectively.

- The covid-bivalent vaccinated group had a statistically significantly higher infection rate than the unvaccinated statewide group ($p < 0.0005$) and the unvaccinated group aged 50 and older ($p = .01$). (Covid-bivalent vaccines target the original strain and the omicron variant.)

101.

Adhikaro B, Bednash JS, et al. **Brief research report: impact of vaccination on antibody responses and mortality from severe COVID-19.** *Front Immunol* 2024 Feb 7; 15: 15:1325243.

"The observation of higher mortality rates among vaccinated versus non-vaccinated patients with severe COVID-19 infection and respiratory failure is a matter of concern."

- Mortality among vaccinated patients was 70% compared with 37% in the non-vaccinated group ($p = 0.0086$). This suggests that among patients with severe infection admitted to the Ohio State University hospital, prior covid vaccination may not always be indicative of protection against mortality.

102.

People who are fully vaccinated against the original strain of Covid-19 are significantly more likely than unvaccinated people to become infected by an alternate strain

"Our results show that there is an increased incidence of [the South African variant] in vaccine breakthrough infections in fully vaccinated individuals [who received the Pfizer-BioNTech vaccine], and increased incidence of [the UK variant] in partially vaccinated individuals."

Kustin T, Harel N, et al. **Evidence for increased breakthrough rates of SARS-CoV-2 variants of concern in BNT162b2 mRNA vaccinated individuals.** *Nat Med* 2021 Aug; 27(8): 1379-84.

- Covid is caused by a coronavirus called severe acute respiratory syndrome coronavirus 2 (SARS-CoV-2).

- Although vaccines were developed to protect against covid, new variants that have the potential to evade these vaccines have emerged.

- In this study, Israeli scientists investigated whether two variants of covid—a South African strain (B.1.351) and a UK strain (B.1.1.7)—are able to overcome the effectiveness of the Pfizer-BioNTech covid vaccine.

- Fully vaccinated people who contracted covid at least one week after the second dose were compared with unvaccinated controls. The prevalence rate of the South African variant was 8 times higher in fully vaccinated versus unvaccinated individuals, 5.4% versus 0.7% (odds ratio, OR = 8.0).

- This study also found that the UK variant was significantly more able to infect partially vaccinated versus unvaccinated individuals (OR = 2.4).

- The breakthrough cases observed in this study (that is, people who contracted covid despite being fully vaccinated) might be due to immune evasion of both strains, or the ability of the UK variant to create higher viral loads.

103.

Newly emerging covid variants are likely to evade existing and future vaccines

"We anticipate that when most of the population is vaccinated, vaccine-resistant mutations will become a more viable mechanism for viral evolution."

Wang R, Chen J, et al. **Emerging vaccine-breakthrough SARS-CoV-2 variants.** *ACS Infect Dis* 2022 Mar 11; 8(3): 546-556.

- To combat covid, several vaccines that mainly target the viral spike (S) proteins were developed. However, mutations on the S gene have led to more infectious variants and vaccine breakthrough infections. These pose a challenge to long-term prevention and control of covid outbreaks.

- A surge of covid infections is being driven by new variants. The molecular mechanism underlying this surge is elusive due to the existence of more than 28,000 unique mutations on the covid spike (S) protein.

- In this paper, scientists integrate the genotyping of more than 1 million covid genomes isolated from patients, tens of thousands of mutational data points, 130 human antibodies, topological data analysis, and deep learning to reveal covid evolution processes and forecast emerging vaccine-escape variants.

- The authors show that infectivity strengthening mutations were the principal mode for viral evolution, while vaccine-escape mutations become a dominant viral evolutionary mechanism within highly vaccinated populations.

- The authors analyzed emerging vaccine-breakthrough co-mutations (multiple mutations emerging concurrently) in 20 highly vaccinated countries, including the US and UK, to identify variants with a high chance of widespread growth.

- The authors predict which emerging co-variants will escape existing vaccines. The ability to accurately forecast emerging covid variants is crucial for the design of novel mutation-proof vaccines and monoclonal antibodies.

- The most dangerous future covid variants will be co-mutations that combine infectivity strengthening mutations with antibody disruptive mutations.

104.

Low social cohesion is predictive of poor antibody response to covid vaccination

"In a population-based study from the UK, we found, for the first time, that people who reported lower social cohesion had poorer antibody response to a single shot of the [covid] vaccine and this was also associated with non-neutralizing antibody protections levels."

Gallagher S, Howard S, et al. **Social cohesion and loneliness are associated with the antibody response to COVID-19 vaccination.** *Brain Behav Immun* 2022 Jul; 103: 179-85.

- In this study, the authors investigated whether social cohesion and loneliness are associated with antibody response to covid vaccination.

- After controlling for variables, lower social cohesion, but not loneliness, was found to be significantly associated with a lower antibody response.

- Individuals that had a lower level of agreement with the statement 'People in this neighborhood can be trusted' had non-neutralizing antibodies to covid vaccination ($p = .03$).

- Although mistrust may negatively affect antibody response to covid vaccination, it may be protective against viral infection due to less social contact and pathogen avoidance.

- This study showed that vaccine efficacy is influenced by the recipient's psychosocial attitudes. If these tendencies are amendable, they could act as vaccine adjuvants.

105.

Ivermectin is protective against covid infections, hospitalizations, and death

"Regular use of ivermectin as a prophylactic agent was associated with significantly reduced COVID-19 infection, hospitalization, and mortality rates."

Kerr L, Cadegiani FA, et al. **Ivermectin prophylaxis used for COVID-19: a citywide, prospective, observational study of 223,128 subjects using propensity score matching.** *Cureus* 2022 Mar 24; 14(3): c61.

- In Itajaí, Brazil, a citywide covid prevention program using ivermectin was implemented. A total of 159,561 subjects were included in the analysis.

- Regular ivermectin users had a significant 44% reduction in covid infections, a 67% reduction in hospitalizations, and a 70% reduction in covid mortality.

- The authors recommend that ivermectin be considered as a preventive strategy, especially for people at higher risk of complications from covid.

106.

Kerr L, Baldi F, et al. **Regular use of ivermectin as prophylaxis for COVID-19 led up to a 92% reduction in COVID-19 mortality rate in a dose-response manner: results of a prospective observational study of a strictly controlled population of 88,012 subjects.** *Cureus* 2022 Aug 31; 14(8): e28624.

"The regular use of ivermectin decreased hospitalization for COVID-19 by 100% [and] mortality by 92% when compared to non-users."

- Ivermectin was optionally prescribed in a dose of 0.2 mg/kg/day for two consecutive days, every 15 days to participants who presented without symptoms of covid. Regular users, irregular users, and non-users were compared.

- There were no hospitalizations for any of the regular users. Non-use increased the mortality rate 12.5-fold. With higher ivermectin intake, there were greater reductions in all undesirable covid outcomes, a dose-response effect.

107.

Ivermectin prevents covid and reduces the risk of death

"The findings indicate with moderate certainty that ivermectin treatment in COVID-19 provides a significant survival benefit. Health professionals should strongly consider its use, in both treatment and prophylaxis."

Bryant A, Lawrie TA, et al. **Ivermectin for prevention and treatment of COVID-19 infection: a systematic review, meta-analysis, and trial sequential analysis to inform clinical guidelines.** *Am J Ther* 2021 Jun 21; 28(4): e434-e460.

- This review of 24 randomized controlled trials comprising 3406 participants assessed the efficacy of ivermectin treatment among people with covid, and as a preventative.

- A meta-analysis of 15 studies found that ivermectin treatment reduced the risk of death by an average of 62% compared with no ivermectin treatment.

- Three studies found that ivermectin prophylaxis among healthcare workers likely reduces the risk of covid infection by an average of 86%.

108.

Ragó Z, Tóth B, et al. **Results of a systematic review and meta-analysis of early studies on ivermectin in SARS-CoV-2 infection.** *Geroscience* 2023 Aug; 45(4): 2179-93.

"Ivermectin has significantly reduced the time to viral clearance in mild to moderate COVID-19 diseases compared to control groups."

- This meta-analysis utilized three studies involving 382 patients to assess the efficacy of ivermectin in covid viral clearance.

- Patients treated with ivermectin cleared the virus 5.74 days sooner than control groups ($p = 0.036$).

109.

Several medical treatments for covid reduce severity of disease and save lives

"For ICU-based critically ill patients, corticosteroids reduced mortality from randomized controlled trial evidence; high-dose intravenous immunoglobulin, ivermectin, and tocilizumab may be associated with reduced mortality when including observational data."

Kim MS, An MH, et al. **Comparative efficacy and safety of pharmacological interventions for the treatment of COVID-19: a systematic review and network meta-analysis.** *PLoS Med* 2020 Dec 30; 17(12): e1003501.

* The authors reviewed 110 studies and 47 medications in 49,569 covid patients to measure viral clearance, progression to severe disease, and mortality.

* For moderate and severe patients hospitalized in non-intensive care units (ICU), corticosteroids, remdesivir, and convalescent plasma reduced the risk of severe pneumonia, admission to ICU, and mechanical ventilation.

* For critically ill patients hospitalized in ICU, corticosteroids, high-dose intravenous immunoglobulin, and ivermectin, significantly lowered mortality.

* Hydroxychloroquine did not reduce progression to severe disease.

110.

Cheng Q, Zhao G, et al. **Comparative efficacy and safety of pharmacological interventions for severe COVID-19 patients: an updated network meta-analysis of 48 randomized controlled trials.** *Medicine (Baltimore)* 2022 Oct 14; 101(41): e30998.

* The authors reviewed 48 randomized controlled trials with 9147 participants to evaluate the efficacy and safety of medications for severe covid infection.

* This paper showed that 12 medications, including ivermectin, intravenous immunoglobulin, convalescent plasma, and remdesivir, were effective at treating severe covid patients and protective against all-cause mortality.

111.

Prior covid infections are highly protective against reinfections from new variants

"Our study's key results indicate that natural infection occurring early in the pandemic produced significant protective benefit against future disease and severe COVID-19 for at least three to six months."

Rick AM, Laurens MB, et al. **Risk of COVID-19 after natural infection or vaccination.** *EbioMedicine* 2023 Oct; 96: 104799.

- This study assessed the protective benefit of a previous covid infection versus vaccine-associated immunity against contracting covid from new variants during a three-to-six month follow-up period.

- A total of 131,306 individuals from several nations were included in the analysis. Covid vaccine clinical trials associated with Moderna, AstraZeneca, Janssen, and Novavax were analyzed.

- Participants were placed into four groups: 1) no previous covid infection and no vaccine, 2) previous infection and no vaccine, 3) no previous infection plus vaccine, and 4) previous infection plus vaccine.

- During the three-to-six month follow-up period, individuals who had previously contracted covid had a 92% decreased risk of contracting a covid infection compared to those who had no prior covid infection (hazard ratio, HR = 0.08).

- This study suggests that mild and/or asymptomatic covid infections may still provide substantial protection, compared to vaccine-induced immunity, against future covid infections.

- Covid infection prior to study enrollment provided significant protection against reinfection during follow-up of the four clinical trials.

- Covid infections that occurred prior to 14 days after the second vaccine doses were administered were not counted.

- Several of the authors received unrelated grants and other forms of payment from vaccine manufacturers, WHO, and the Gates Foundation.

112.

Natural immunity is more robust against covid infections and hospitalizations than vaccine-induced immunity

"Our study showed that natural immunity offers stronger and longer-lasting protection against infection, symptoms, and hospitalization compared to vaccine-induced immunity."

Uusküla A, Pisarev H, et al. **Risk of SARS-CoV-2 infection and hospitalization in individuals with natural, vaccine-induced and hybrid immunity: a retrospective population-based cohort study from Estonia.** *Sci Rep* 2023 Nov 21; 13(1): 20347.

- This study compared covid infections and hospitalizations in people with natural, vaccine-induced, and hybrid immunity.

- There were 94,982 people in the natural immunity cohort, 47,342 in the hybrid cohort, and 254,920 in the vaccine group.

- Individuals with natural immunity were five times less likely than those with no immunity to become infected during the Delta period (incidence rate, IR per 100 = 3.8 vs 20.1). Natural immunity against hospitalization was substantial in the Delta (adjusted hazard ratio = 0.05) and Omicron (aHR = 0.10) periods.

- Naturally immune females were two times less likely to be hospitalized than naturally immune men, and increasing age significantly contributed to the risk of covid hospitalization.

- Individuals with hybrid immunity were less likely to become infected than those with natural immunity during the Delta period, but not during the Omicron period. Covid hospitalization was rare in this group.

- Individuals with vaccine-induced immunity were nearly five times more likely than those with natural immunity to become infected during the Delta period (aHR = 4.90). During Omicrion, they were 13% more likely. They were at increased risk of hospitalization during the Delta period as well (aHR = 7.19).

Covid Vaccine and Cardiovascular Events

Cardiovascular adverse events occur after receipt of the covid vaccine. For example, myocarditis (inflammation of the heart muscle) and pericarditis (inflammation of the outer lining of the heart) are significantly more likely to occur up to four weeks after covid vaccination. Young, healthy males 12 to 29 years of age are most affected. Females are most likely to have persisting symptoms after mRNA covid vaccination.

Atrial fibrillation, cardiac arrhythmia, thombocytopenia, and death are also possible after covid vaccination. In 12 to 39 year olds, the risk of a cerebral venous thrombosis (a blood clot in the brain) is 16 times greater in the 4-13 days after a covid vaccine compared to an unvaccinated population. Loss of vision due to a retinal blood clot is also possible after covid vaccination.

113.

Covid vaccination significantly increases the risk of severe heart damage

"These findings raise concerns regarding vaccine-induced undetected severe cardiovascular side-effects and underscore the already established causal relationship between vaccines and myocarditis, a frequent cause of unexpected cardiac arrest in young individuals."

Sun CLF, Jaffe E, Levi R. **Increased emergency cardiovascular events among under-40 population in Israel during vaccine rollout and third COVID-19 wave.** *Sci Rep* 2022 Apr 28; 12(1): 6978.

- This study used data from Israel's national emergency medical services (EMS) to determine whether covid-19 infections and/or vaccinations are associated with excessive EMS calls for cardiac arrest and acute coronary syndrome.

- This study compared the volume of EMS calls during three time periods: 1) the pre-pandemic or baseline period (2019), 2) the pandemic period (2020), and 3) the vaccination period (Jan-May 2021).

- Regarding people aged 16-39, the volume of EMS calls for cardiac arrest and acute coronary syndrome increased by 25% during the covid-19 vaccine rollout (Jan-May 2021) compared with the same months during the pre-pandemic (2019) and pandemic (2020) periods.

- EMS calls for cardiac arrest and acute coronary syndrome started increasing by early Jan 2021 and seemed to track closely with the second vaccine dose.

- For cardiac arrest, there was no statistical difference in EMS call volume in 2020 (the pandemic period) as compared to 2019 (the pre-pandemic period). The graphs in this paper highlight the lack of association between covid *infections* and EMS calls for cardiac arrest and acute coronary syndrome.

- For adults aged 40 and older, EMS calls for cardiac arrest and acute coronary syndrome were also significantly higher during the vaccination period.

- The authors recommend advising covid-vaccinated patients experiencing heart symptoms to avoid strenuous physical activity and seek medical care.

114.

Cardiac abnormalities in teens, caused by covid vaccination, persist for months

"In a cohort of adolescents with COVID-19 mRNA vaccine-related myopericarditis, a large portion have persistent LGE abnormalities, raising concerns for potential longer-term effects."

Schauer J, Buddhe S, et al. **Persistent cardiac magnetic resonance imaging findings in a cohort of adolescents with post-coronavirus disease 2019 mRNA vaccine myopericarditis.** *J Pediatr* 2022 Jun; 245; 233-37.

- Myopericarditis has become an important adverse event caused by covid-19 mRNA vaccination, especially in adolescent males. Patients typically develop chest pain and an elevated serum troponin level (evidence of a heart attack) 2-4 days following the second dose of covid vaccination.

- In this paper, 16 adolescents who were diagnosed with myopericarditis after receiving a second dose of the covid-19 mRNA vaccine were medically evaluated with a cardiac MRI within 1 week of initial symptoms and a follow-up MRI 3-8 months later.

- The initial cardiac MRIs were all abnormal. Other common symptoms were an abnormal ECG, fever, and shortness of breath.

- Although there was a significant decrease in LGE (late gadolinium enhancement) during follow-up, eleven patients (68.8%) had persistent LGE, which previous studies have shown is a predictor of adverse cardiovascular outcomes, including all-cause death.

- More studies are required to determine the ultimate clinical significance of persistent cardiac MRI abnormalities in patients with covid-19 vaccine-related myopericarditis.

115.

Myocarditis and pericarditis are significantly more likely to occur up to four weeks after covid vaccination

"We may speculate that mRNA SARS-CoV-2 vaccines, like other vaccines, act as a non-specific trigger that in a limited number of susceptible subjects may activate the inflammatory pathways inducing myocarditis and pericarditis."

Conte E, Leoni O, et al. **Incidence of myocarditis and pericarditis considered as separate clinical events over the years and post-SARS-CoV2 vaccination in adults and children.** *Eur J Intern Med* 2023 Sep; 115: 140-42.

- This study assessed the association between covid vaccination and myocarditis and pericarditis using health databases from Italy.

- The authors compared patients who were diagnosed with myocarditis and/or pericarditis during the first 28 days after covid vaccination (the high-risk period) to those who experience these ailments outside the high risk period.

- Recipients of the Moderna covid vaccine were six time more likely to develop myocarditis during the high-risk period, even after adjusting for potential confounders (incidence rate ratio, IRR = 6.76). Pfizer vaccine recipients were twice as likely to develop myocarditis after vaccination (IRR = 2.48).

- Recipients of Moderna and Pfizer vaccines also had significantly higher rates of pericarditis. The prevalence of pericarditis in patients younger than 30 years of age was especially higher after covid vaccination ($p < 0.0001$).

- This study found a significantly higher risk of both myocarditis and pericarditis during the first 28 days after Modernal and Pfizer mRNA covid vaccines.

116.

mRNA covid vaccines increase the risk of myocarditis and pericarditis

"Vaccination program strategies, such as age-based product considerations and longer interdose intervals, may reduce the risk of myocarditis or pericarditis following receipt of mRNA vaccines."

Buchan SA, Seo CY, et al. **Epidemiology of myocarditis and pericarditis following mRNA vaccination by vaccine product, schedule, and interdose interval among adolescents and adults in Ontario, Canada.** *JAMA Netw Open* 2022 Jun 1; 5(6): e2218505.

- This study examined rates of reported myocarditis or pericarditis following mRNA covid vaccination using data from Ontario, Canada's vaccine registry and vaccine safety surveillance system.

- Of 297 reports of myocarditis or pericarditis, 76.8% occurred in males, and 69.7% occurred after the second vaccine dose.

- Males 18-24 years of age had the highest rate of myocarditis or pericarditis following a second dose of Moderna's mRNA vaccine: 299.5 cases per 1 million doses. Male children 12-17 years of age had the second highest rate.

- Rates of myocarditis or pericarditis were significantly higher when the second dose was given within 30 or fewer days after the first dose, as compared to vaccine recipients who waited at least 8 weeks to receive their second dose.

- The median time to symptom onset was 3 days post-vaccination. For adverse events after a second dose, 86.9% occurred within 7 days of vaccination. Nearly all events (97.6%) required an emergency department visit.

- Rates of myocarditis or pericarditis after a second dose were significantly higher in recipients of the Moderna versus Pfizer covid vaccine: 6 time higher for males and 9 times higher for females 18-24 years of age.

- Mixing Pfizer's vaccine for dose 1 and Moderna's for dose 2 was associated with higher adverse events than a Moderna vaccine for doses 1 and 2.

117.

Males 12 to 24 years old have the worst rates of myocarditis after mRNA covid vaccination

"Cases of myocarditis reported after COVID-19 vaccination were typically diagnosed within days of vaccination."

Oster ME, Shay DK, et al. **Myocarditis cases reported after mRNA-based COVID-19 vaccination in the US from December 2020 to August 2021.** *JAMA* 2022 Jan 25; 327(4): 331-340.

- In this study, CDC-sponsored scientists analyzed the Vaccine Adverse Event Reporting System (VAERS) for reports of myocarditis that occurred within seven days after mRNA covid vaccines were administered to US individuals 12 years of age and older.

- Rates were highest after the second Pfizer vaccine in male teens 16 to 17 years old: 105.9 cases of myocarditis per million doses. Males aged 12 to 15 years developed myocarditis at 70.7 cases per million doses. Young men aged 18 to 24 years: 56.3 cases per million doses of the Moderna vaccine.

- Myocarditis rates were highest in females 16-17 years after the second dose of Pfizer's covid vaccine: 11 cases per million doses. In women 25 to 29 years: 8.2 cases per million Moderna doses. In women, 18 to 24 years of age: 6.9 cases per million doses. In females 12 to 15 years: 6.4 cases per million doses.

- Males 12 to 15 years of age were 133 times more likely than expected to develop myocarditis after receipt of a second dose of Pfizer's covid vaccine. Females 12 to 15 years of age were 37 times more likely than expected to develop myocarditis after receipt of a second dose of Pfizer's covid vaccine.

- Individuals who developed myocarditis after covid vaccination should defer additional doses of mRNA-based covid vaccines.

- VAERS reports of myocarditis had a high verification rate indicating that under-reporting is likely. Thus, actual rates of myocarditis per million doses are probably higher than indicated in this study.

118.

Male adolescents have the highest rates of myocarditis and pericarditis after covid vaccination

"There is a significant increase in the risk of acute myocarditis/ pericarditis following Comirnaty vaccination among Chinese male adolescents, especially after the second dose."

Chua GT, Kwan MYW, et al. **Epidemiology of acute myocarditis/ pericarditis in Hong Kong adolescents following Comirnaty vaccin- ation.** *Clin Infect Dis* 2022 Sep 10; 75(4): 673-81.

- Scientists studied the characteristics and incidence of acute myocarditis/ pericarditis among Hong Kong adolescents 12 to 17 years of age following mRNA covid vaccination (Comirnaty vaccine).

- During approximately three months in 2021 (including a 14-day follow-up period), 33 adolescents developed myocarditis/pericarditis following covid vaccination. In total, 88% were male and 12% were female. Of all cases, 82% occurred after the second vaccine dose.

- The overall incidence of myocarditis/pericarditis was 185 per million persons vaccinated, and 212 per million persons vaccinated after the second dose. Among male adolescents, the incidence after the second dose was 373 per million persons vaccinated.

- Compared to the background rate of acute myocarditis/pericarditis from 2011 to 2020 (prior to covid vaccines) there were significantly higher incidence rate differences in vaccinated adolescents, consistent with the main findings.

- The US CDC estimated 40.6 cases of myocarditis/pericarditis after mRNA covid vaccination per million second doses among males 12 to 29 years old, much lower than the rates found in this study.

- Health professionals and mRNA covid vaccine recipients should be attentive to symptoms of myocarditis and pericarditis.

119.

Males 16 to 29 years of age have the worst rates of myocarditis after Pfizer's mRNA covid vaccination

"The diagnosis of myocarditis occurred throughout the post-vaccination period, but there appeared to be an increase approximately 3 to 5 days after the second vaccine dose."

Witberg G, Barda N, et al. **Myocarditis after covid-19 vaccination in a large health care organization.** *NEJM* 2021 Dec 2; 385(23): 2132-39.

- The authors searched the database of Israel's largest health care organization for diagnoses of myocarditis in patients who had received at least one dose of Pfizer's mRNA covid vaccine. They analyzed the incidence of myocarditis up to 42 days after the first vaccine dose.

- The highest incidence of myocarditis was in males 16 to 29 years old: 106.9 cases per one million vaccinated persons.

120.

Pueyo PP, Ruberte EG, et al. **Vaccine-carditis study: Spanish multicenter registry of inflammatory heart disease after COVID-19 vaccination.** *Clin Res Cardiol* 2024 Feb; 113(2): 223-234.

"Inflammatory heart disease after vaccination against SARS-CoV-2 predominantly affects young men in the 1st week after the second dose of RNA-m vaccine."

- In this Spanish study, 139 cases of inflammatory heart disease (myocarditis or pericarditis) after covid vaccination were identified.

- Eighty-one percent of cases were in young males.

- Most cases were detected in the first week after receipt of an mRNA covid vaccine, the majority after the second dose.

121.

Females are more likely to have persisting symptoms after mRNA covid vaccine-related myocarditis

"In our observational study a relevant proportion of patients with confirmed vaccine-related myocarditis reported persisting complaints. While mRNA vaccine-related myocarditis usually affects young males, these patients with persisting symptoms were predominantly females and older."

Schroth D, Garg R, et al. **Predictors of persistent symptoms after mRNA SARS-CoV-2 vaccine-related myocarditis (myovacc registry).** *Front Cardiovasc Med* 2023 Jun 21; 10: 1204232.

- Researchers evaluated 59 patients from Canada and Germany diagnosed with acute myocarditis after mRNA covid vaccination. The most common symptoms at baseline were chest pain and dyspnea (labored breathing).

- Fifty-one of the 59 patients (86%) were admitted to the hospital; 29% were admitted to the ICU. ST segment changes in the electrocardiogram were found in 37%, while 100% had elevated levels of hs-troponin-T (which aids in the diagnosis of myocardial infarction).

- In 24% of the patients, symptoms of chest pain, dyspnea, fatigue, and palpitations persisted for a median interval of seven months.

- Most myocarditis cases occurred in young males (mean age = 29 years) after the second dose of mRNA vaccination.

- Although young males are most affected by myocarditis after vaccination, patients with persisting symptoms were predominantly older females.

- The initial severity of myocarditis was not associated with long-term complaints. Female gender and dyspnea at initial presentation were significant predictors of persistent symptoms.

- There are similarities between persisting symptoms after mRNA vaccine-related myocarditis and long-covid.

122.

Rates of myocarditis were higher in covid vaccinated versus unvaccinated people, and in vaccinated people versus pre-pandemic controls

"On the basis of data from an Israeli national database, the incidence of myocarditis after two doses of the [Pfizer] mRNA vaccine was low but higher than the incidence among unvaccinated persons and among historical controls."

Mevorach D, Anis E, et al. **Myocarditis after BNT162b2 mRNA vaccine against Covid-19 in Israel.** *N Engl J Med* 2021 Dec 2; 385(23): 2140-49.

- The Israeli Ministry of Health initiated active surveillance of all cases of myocarditis after Pfizer mRNA covid vaccination from December 20, 2020 to May 31, 2021. They then calculated the standardized incidence ratio (IR) and rate ratio (RR) after the first and second vaccine dose.

- The IR for 16-19 year olds (as compared with pre-pandemic expected incidence) after the second dose was 13.60 in males and 6.74 in females. The IR for 20-24 year olds after the second dose was 10.76 in females and 8.53 in males.

- The RR for 16-19 year olds within 30 days after the second dose was 8.96 in males and 2.95 in females. The RR for 20-24 year olds after the second dose was 7.56 in females and 6.13 in males.

- When follow-up was restricted to 7 days after the second vaccine dose rather than 30 days, the RR for males 16 to 19 years old was much higher: 31.90.

- Myocarditis after the second dose of Pfizer's covid vaccine occurred in males 16 to 19 years old at a rate of 150.7 cases per one million vaccinated persons. In males 20 to 24 years old, the rate was 108.6 cases per million.

- In this study, rates of myocarditis were higher in a) covid vaccinated versus unvaccinated people, and b) covid vaccinated people versus pre-pandemic (or historical) controls.

123.

Chest pain, myocarditis and death are possible after covid vaccination

"In teenagers who present with chest pain after COVID-19 mRNA vaccination, confirmed myocarditis is uncommon. However, myocardial abnormalities on [a cardiac MRI] might occur frequently."

Park CH, Yang J, et al. **Characteristics of teenagers presenting with chest pain after COVID-19 mRNA vaccination.** *J Clin Med* 2023 Jun 30; 12(13): 4421.

- The authors evaluated laboratory results of 61 teenagers, 13 to 19 years, who had echocardiography and cardiac magnetic resonance imaging (CMR) for chest pain after covid mRNA vaccination.

- Among the 61 patients with chest pain following covid vaccination, only two (3.3%) were diagnosed with myocarditis. Yet, on CMR, 24 (39.3%) showed mild myocardial abnormalities, 22 (36.1%) showed myocardial edema, and 19 (31.1%) were found to have a myocardial injury.

- Of all 61 patients, 43% and 57% developed chest pain after the first and second vaccine doses, respectively. Chest pain developed within 3 to 7 days after vaccination and continued for about 7 to 10 days. Teens with continuous chest pain after covid vaccination may be vulnerable to a myocardial injury.

124.

Hulscher N, Hodkinson R, et al. **Autopsy findings in cases of fatal COVID-19 vaccine-induced myocarditis.** *ESC Heart Fail* 2024 Jan 14: 10.1002/ehf2.14680.

"We identified a series of myocarditis-related deaths after COVID-19 vaccination, confirmed with autopsies, to provide...a more comprehensive understanding of fatal COVID-19 vaccine-induced myocarditis."

- Six days was the average time between the last covid vaccination until death. The findings in this paper suggest that "there is a high likelihood of a causal link" between covid vaccination and death from myocarditis.

125.

The risk of myopericarditis after mRNA covid vaccination is much higher than that reported to US vaccine advisory committees

"Complete case estimates are essential when modeling risk and benefit for wide-scale vaccine implementation and booster doses in younger age groups."

Sharff KA, Dancoes DM, et al. **Risk of myopericarditis following COVID-19 mRNA vaccination in a large integrated health system: a comparison of completeness and timeliness of two methods.** *Pharmacoepidemiol Drug Saf* 2022 Aug; 31(8): 921-25.

- The authors identified a cohort of 12 to 39 year-old patients who received at least one dose of Pfizer's or Moderna's mRNA covid vaccine. They followed them for up to 30 days after their second covid vaccine to determine their risk of myocarditis, pericarditis, or myopericarditis.

- In males 12 to 17 and 18 to 24 years old, the estimated risks of myopericarditis are 377 and 537 cases per million second covid vaccine doses, respectively.

- The authors calculated the number of myopericarditis cases following covid vaccination by searching text descriptions in an integrated health system. Their estimated case numbers are much higher than those derived from the Vaccine Safety Datalink (VSD) methodology, which has several flaws.

- The VSD excluded myocarditis, unspecified (ICD code I51.4) resulting in missed diagnoses. The VSD also used a 21-day cutoff, instead of a 30-day cutoff used by the authors, which allowed them to identify additional cases. And the VSDs lag in data submission may cause inaccurate case counts.

- The authors' estimated incidence of myopericarditis following covid vaccination is similar to case counts reported in studies from Israel and Hong Kong but higher than that reported to US vaccine advisory committees.

- The authors' methodology (versus VSD-derived estimates) identified about twice as many cases of myopericarditis following mRNA covid vaccination.

126.

Covid vaccination increases the risk of cardiac-related mortality

"The pooled hazard ratio suggests that COVID-19 vaccination is associated with an increased risk of cardiac-related mortality."

Marchand G, Masoud AT, Medi S. **Risk of all-cause and cardiac-related mortality after vaccination against COVID-19: A meta-analysis of self-controlled case series studies.** *Hum Vaccin Immunother* 2023 Aug 1; 19(2): 2230828.

- The authors investigated all-cause and cardiac-related mortality following covid vaccination.

- Covid vaccination was found to be associated with a significantly increased risk of cardiac-related mortality (hazard ratio, HR = 1.06; p = .007), especially in males: (HR = 1.09; p = .006).

- No relationship was found between covid vaccination and all-cause mortality.

127.

Nakahara T, Iwabuchi Y, et al. **Assessment of myocardial ^{18}F-FDG uptake at PET/CT in asymptomatic SARS-CoV-2-vaccinated and non-vaccinated patients.** *Radiology* 2023 Sep; 308(3): e230743.

- This study tested 700 asymptomatic covid-vaccinated adults to determine if they have silent or hidden changes in heart muscle function.

- The 700 covid-vaccinated and 303 non-vaccinated adults all underwent PET-CT scans. Patients who received their second covid vaccine up to 180 days prior to their scans had significantly higher myocardial ^{18}Fluorine-fluorodeoxy-glucose (^{18}F-FDG) uptake, indicative of abnormal cardiac function.

- Compared to non-vaccinated adults, myocardial ^{18}F-FDG uptake was significantly higher (p < .001) in covid-vaccinated adults regardless of sex, age, or type of mRNA vaccine received.

128.

Atrial fibrillation, a serious heart condition, can occur after mRNA covid vaccination

"We found and analyzed more than 6000 reports describing atrial fibrillation as an adverse event following immunization with anti-COVID-19 vaccines collected in the Eudravigilance database. The majority of the retrieved reports were related to mRNA vaccines."

Ruggiero R, Donniacuo M, et al. **COVID-19 Vaccines and atrial fibrillation: analysis of the post-marketing pharmacovigilance European database.** *Biomedicines* 2023 May 30; 11(6): 1584.

- The authors analyzed cases of atrial fibrillation after covid vaccination reported in the European post-marketing database, Eudravigilance, from 2020 to November 2022. Atrial fibrillation is an irregular, rapid heartbeat that needs proper treatment to prevent stroke.

- Atrial fibrillation required hospitalization in 35% of cases and caused a life-threatening condition in 10% of cases.

- Other cardiac disorders that occurred with atrial fibrillation were myocarditis, pericarditis, palpitations, tachycardia, chest pain, and cardiac failure.

129.

Al-Yafeai Z, Ghoweba M, et al. **Vaccines and atrial fibrillation: a real-world pharmacovigilance study based on Vaccine Adverse Event Reporting System.** *Am J Ther* 2023 Mar-Apr; 30(2): 151-53.

"Our results showed that COVID-19 vaccines reported the most frequent atrial fibrillation (84%) among all other vaccines."

- The authors accessed the VAERS database from 1990 to 2021 to determine the reported incidence of atrial fibrillation following receipt of different vaccines.

- People who received the covid-19 vaccine had a significantly higher risk of developing atrial fibrillation with a reporting odds ratio of 13.18 ($p < 0.0001$).

130.

Cardiac arrhythmia occurs after mRNA covid vaccination

"mRNA vaccines, including Moderna and Pfizer, were associated with a higher incidence ratio rate of arrhythmia than vector-based vaccines."

Abutaleb MH, Makeen HA, et al. **Risks of cardiac arrhythmia associated with COVID-19 vaccination: a systematic review and meta-analysis.** *Vaccines (Basel)* 2023 Jan 3; 11(1): 112.

- The authors systematically reviewed 17 studies to summarize evidence of an association between covid vaccination and cardiac arrhythmia.

- The risk of cardiac arrhythmia occurred at a rate of 7600 per million after Moderna vaccination and 2200 per million after Pfizer vaccination.

131.

Shi A, Tang X, et al. **Cardiac arrhythmia after COVID-19 vaccination versus non-COVID-19 vaccination: a systematic review and meta-analysis.** *Circulation* 2023; 148: A12013.

"The overall risk for arrhythmia after COVID-19 vaccination was...higher in COVID-19 vaccine recipients than in non-COVID-19 vaccine recipients."

- The authors analyzed 36 studies to compare the risk of cardiac arrhythmia after covid vaccination with the risk after non-covid vaccination.

- Cases of arrhythmia were significantly higher after covid vaccination than after non-covid vaccination: 2263 vs. 9.9 cases per million doses ($p < 0.01$).

- Tachyarrhythmia (abnormal rhythms above 100 beats per minute) was also higher after covid vaccination: 4367 vs. 25.8 cases per million doses.

- Arrhythmia was more frequent after the third dose of a covid vaccine: 19,064 cases per million doses.

132.

Thrombocytopenia and death are possible after covid vaccination

"Thrombosis with thrombocytopenia syndrome (TTS) associated with viral vector COVID-19 vaccines, including AstraZeneca vaccine, can result in significant morbidity and mortality."

Tran HA, Deng L, et al. **The clinicopathological features of thrombosis with thrombocytopenia syndrome following ChAdOx1-S (AZD1222) vaccination and case outcomes in Australia: a population-based study.** *Lancet Reg Health West Pac* 2023 Sep 4; 40: 100894.

• Australian scientists identified 170 cases of thrombosis with thrombocytopenia syndrome (TTS) after receipt of an AstraZeneca covid vaccine. TTS is a life-threatening blood clotting disorder of the brain, abdomen, leg, or lung.

• Ninety-six percent of the 170 patients with vaccine-induced TTS were hospitalized (range = 3-13 days), 39% were admitted to intensive care, and 16% required surgical intervention. There were eight deaths (4.7%).

• A higher risk of death was related to a lower platelet count (OR = 1.82), a cerebral or abdominal thrombosis (OR = 5.16), or hemorrhage during admission (OR = 14.82). Of all TTS cases, 71% were either overweight or obese.

133.

Yasmin F, Najeeb H, et al. **Adverse events following COVID-19 mRNA vaccines: a systematic review of cardiovascular complication, thrombosis, and thrombocytopenia.** *Immun Inflamm Dis* 2023 Mar; 11 (3): e807.

"Cardiovascular events such as thrombosis, thrombocytopenia, stroke, and myocarditis frequently occur with the mRNA vaccines."

• This paper analyzed 17,636 people with cardiovascular complications, including 284 deaths, after their covid vaccines. Thrombosis, stroke, myocarditis, and pulmonary embolism were the most frequently reported cardiovascular events.

• More than 80% of deaths occurred after the Pfizer vaccine.

134.

Blood clots in the brain are possible after covid vaccination

"This epidemiological study shows an increased risk of thrombotic episodes and thrombocytopenia in adults under 65 years of age within a month of a first dose of ChAdOx1 [AstraZeneca] vaccine."

Andrews NJ, Stowe J, et al. **Risk of venous thrombotic events and thrombocytopenia in sequential time periods after ChAdOx1 and BNT162b2 COVID-19 vaccines: a national cohort study in England.** *Lancet Reg Health Eur* 2022 Feb; 13: 100260.

- Scientists in England assessed the risk of hospital admissions for a cerebral venous thrombosis (blood clot in the brain) and thrombocytopenia (low blood platelet count) following receipt of an AstraZeneca covid vaccine.

- Compared to an unvaccinated baseline, the risk of a cerebral venous thrombosis (CVT) after a first dose of AstraZeneca's covid vaccine in 15-39 year olds was highest 4-13 days post-vaccination (relative incidence, RI = 16.3, $p <$ 0.0001). This translates to 16.1 cases per million vaccine doses.

- The risk in this age group of a CVT was still high after 28 days (RI = 6.6, $p < 0.0001$). The risk of thrombosis with thrombocytopenia in 15-39 year olds was also highest 4-13 days post-vaccination (RI = 38.2). Other types of venous thrombosis occurred at a rate of 36.3 cases per million doses.

- In 40-64 year olds, the risk of a CVT (RI = 2.8) or thrombocytopenia was highest 14-27 days post-vaccination (RI = 2.8 for each condition, $p = .0001$). Thrombosis with thrombocytopenia occurred at a higher rate (RI = 5.4).

135.

Lu Y, Matuska K, et al. **Stroke after COVID-19 bivalent vaccination among US older adults.** *JAMA* 2024; 331(11): 938-50.

- There was a statistically significant link between the concurrent receipt of the Pfizer covid vaccine plus an adjuvanted influenza vaccine and transient ischemic attack (IRR = 1.35) and nonhemorrhagic stroke (IRR = 1.20).

136.

Blood clots in the brain and other venous thromboembolism events are definite or probable after covid vaccination

"We confirm the relative incidence of cerebral venous thrombosis and other venous thromboembolism events is significantly increased following first dose of ChAdOx1 vaccine."

Shaw RJ, Doyle AJ, et al. **Re-evaluation of the risk of venous thromboembolism after COVID-19 vaccination using haematological criteria.** *Vaccine* 2023 Aug 14; 41(36): 5330-37.

- All cases of severe thrombocytopenia occurred after a first dose of covid vaccine. Severe thrombocytopenia did not occur in the unvaccinated cohort.

- The estimated number of vaccine-induced cases of cerebral venous thrombosis in 18-39 year olds after a first dose of AstraZeneca's covid vaccine is 95.19 per million doses. In 18-64 year olds, other types of venous thromboembolism (e.g., pulmonary, deep vein) occurred at a rate of 76.52 per million doses.

137.

Li J, Wang Y, et al. **Risk assessment of retinal vascular occlusion after COVID-19 vaccination.** *NPJ Vaccines* 2023 May 2; 8(1): 64.

"We demonstrated a higher risk and incidence rate of retinal vascular occlusion following COVID-19 vaccination, after adjusting for potential confounding factors."

- The authors investigated the risk of retinal vascular occlusion (blurry vision or loss of vision) after covid vaccination.

- The authors compared 739,066 covid-vaccinated and unvaccinated people.

- Vaccinated individuals were twice as likely to develop all forms of retinal vascular occlusion within two years after vaccination (HR = 2.19).

Covid Vaccine and Paralysis
(GBS and Bell's Palsy)

Guillain-Barré syndrome (GBS) and Bells Palsy (facial paralysis) often occur after covid vaccination. Vector-based covid vaccines, like Johnson & Johnson's Janssen or AstraZeneca's Vaxzevria, seem most prone to causing these adverse events. According to Lehmann, GBS cases occur at a rate four times higher than expected in all age groups 3-42 days after the Janssen vaccine and three times higher than expected after Vaxzevria. In the ≥80 year age group GBS is 16 times higher than expected. Hanson put the incidence rate of GBS at 324 per million person-years in the 1 to 21 day period following Janssen's covid vaccine, significantly higher than the background rate.

La found that without information on the dose of mRNA vaccination, the incidence rate of post-vaccination Bell's palsy is 310.8 per million persons. Shibli used Israel's largest healthcare provider's database to assess the association between Pfizer's mRNA covid vaccine and Bell's palsy. In the 16 and older age group, the risk of Bell's palsy within 21 days after the first vaccine dose is 50.9 cases per one million people vaccinated. In vaccinated patients with a previous history of Bell's palsy, the risk of Bell's palsy within 21 days after the first vaccine dose is 528.6 cases per million people vaccinated.

138.

Vector-based covid vaccines increase the risk of Guillain-Barré syndrome

"Guillain-Barré syndrome could be an adverse event after vaccination with vector-based COVID-19 vaccines."

Lehmann HC, Oberle D, et al. **Rare cases of Guillain-Barré syndrome after COVID-19 vaccination, Germany, December 2020 to August 2021.** *Euro Surveill* 2023 Jun; 28(24): 2200744.

- This German study analyzed 156 cases of Guillain-Barré syndrome (GBS) that occurred after covid vaccination.

- GBS cases occurred at a rate four times higher than expected in all age groups (standardized morbidity ratio, SMR = 4.16) 3-42 days after the Janssen covid vaccine was administered, and three times higher than expected after Astra-Zeneca's Vaxzevria (SMR = 3.10).

- After the Janssen vaccine, rates of GBS were even higher in the 40-49, 60-69, and ≥80 year age groups: SMRs = 5.55, 6.76, and 16.82, respectively.

139.

Shao S, Wang C, et al. **Guillain-Barré syndrome associated with COVID-19 vaccination.** *Emerg Infect Dis* 2021 Dec; 27(12): 3175-78.

"Our findings highlight the need for vigilance in patients with neurologic symptoms after COVID-19 vaccination."

- Taiwanese researchers reviewed 39 cases of GBS that occurred within two weeks following covid vaccination. Initial symptoms included myalgia, paraparesis, quadriparesis, paresthesia, and facial palsy.

- The GBS rate after covid vaccination ranged from 1.8 to 53.2 cases per one million doses.

140.

Guillain-Barré syndrome is a recognized risk after vector-based covid vaccines

"Emerging data support a temporal association between GBS and adenovirus-vector COVID-19 vaccines."

Osowicki J, Morgan HJ, et al. **Guillain-Barré syndrome temporally associated with COVID-19 vaccines in Victoria, Australia.** *Vaccine* 2022 Dec 12; 40(52): 7579-85.

- Australian researchers reviewed 41 cases of GBS that occurred within six weeks after covid vaccination, with a median onset of 14 days.

- Regarding AstraZeneca's covid vaccine, there were 35 reports following the first dose, translating to 18.5 cases per million doses.

141.

Ha J, Park S, et al. **Real-world data on the incidence and risk of Guillain-Barré syndrome following SARS-CoV-2 vaccination: a prospective surveillance study.** *Sci Rep* 2023 Mar 7; 13(1): 3773.

"The initial dose of viral-vector based vaccine and later doses of mRNA-based vaccine were associated with GBS, respectively."

- The South Korean government cooperated with the Korean Disease Control and Prevention Agency to estimate the incidence rate of Guillain-Barré syndrome (GBS) after covid vaccination.

- For mRNA and vector-based covid vaccines, GBS occurred at a rate of 0.8 and 4.49 cases per million doses, respectively.

- GBS occurred most often after the first dose of the vector-based covid vaccine, and after the second and third doses of the mRNA vaccines.

142.

Health officials found that vaccination against covid increases the risk of GBS

"In this retrospective cohort study, we found evidence for increased risks of Guillain-Barré syndrome within 21- and 42-day intervals after Ad26.COV2.S [Janssen/Johnson & Johnson] vaccination."

Abara WE, Gee J, et al. **Reports of Guillain-Barré syndrome after COVID-19 vaccination in the United States.** *JAMA Netw Open* 2023 Feb 1; 6(2): e2253845.

- This study, conducted by the CDC and FDA, compared Guillain-Barré syndrome (GBS) reporting patterns after covid vaccination in the United States.

- The authors identified 912 GBS reports in VAERS. After review of associated medical records, 295 (32.3%) of the total reports were verified.

- Within 42 days of vaccination, there were 4.07 GBS reports per one million doses of the Janssen (Johnson & Johnson) covid vaccine—12 and 9 times more frequently reported than Pfizer's and Moderna's covid vaccines.

143.

LeVu S, Bertrand M, et al. **Risk of Guillain-Barré syndrome following COVID-19 vaccines: a nationwide self-controlled case series study.** *Neurology* 2023 Nov 21; 101(21): e2094-e2102.

"We found increased risks of Guillain-Barré syndrome following the first administration of [AstraZeneca] and [Janssen] vaccines."

- Health officials used the French National Health Data System and covid vaccine database to estimate rates of GBS within 6 weeks post-vaccination.

- There were 6.5 and 5.7 attributable GBS cases per million persons after the first dose of the AstraZeneca and Janssen vaccines, respectively.

- After the second dose of the mRNA Moderna vaccine, the relative incidence of GBS in the 12-49 year age group was significantly high: (RI = 2.6).

144.

Guillain-Barré syndrome, myocarditis, pericarditis, thrombocytopenia, and death are possible after Janssen covid vaccination

"Our review confirmed previously established safety risks for thrombosis with thrombocytopenia syndrome and Guillain-Barré syndrome, and identified a potential safety concern for myocarditis."

Woo EJ, Gee J, et al. **Post-authorization safety surveillance of Ad.26. COV2.S vaccine: reports to the Vaccine Adverse Event Reporting System and V-safe, February 2021–February 2022.** *Vaccine* 2023 July 5; 41(30): 4422-30.

- FDA and CDC scientists reviewed VAERS data and V-safe (a vaccine safety monitoring system) for adverse events after Johnson & Johnson's Janssen covid vaccine during the first year of the U.S. covid vaccination program.

- The estimated observed-to-expected rate ratio of GBS post-vaccination was 4.18, corresponding to an absolute rate increase of 63.6 per million person-years.

- Among adults 18-29 years of age, verified cases of myopericarditis within seven days of Janssen covid vaccination occurred at an observed-to-expected rate ratio of RR = 102.4 per million.

- In total, 8245 reported adverse events were serious, with 1528 deaths. The most common causes of death post-vaccination were covid, diseases of the heart, and cerebrovascular diseases.

- All reports of thrombosis with thrombocytopenia syndrome (TTS) meeting the CDC case definition, and immune thrombocytopenia (ITP) with a documented platelet count, were serious.

- Other serious conditions that occurred post-vaccination include covid, myopericarditis, pregnancy loss, seizure, stroke, and Bell's palsy.

- Fact sheets were updated to include warnings about myocarditis, pericarditis, TTS, GBS, and other adverse events that may occur post-vaccination.

145.

The CDC's Vaccine Safety Datalink database confirmed that Johnson & Johnson's covid vaccine causes Guillain-Barré syndrome

"In this cohort study of COVID-19 vaccines, the incidence of Guillain-Barré syndrome was elevated after receiving the Janssen (Johnson & Johnson) vaccine."

Hanson KE, Goddard K, et al. **Incidence of Guillain-Barré syndrome after COVID-19 vaccination in the Vaccine Safety Datalink.** *JAMA Netw Open* 2022 Apr 1; 5(4): e228879.

- This study investigated the incidence of Guillain-Barré syndrome after Janssen (Johnson & Johnson) vector-based versus mRNA (Pfizer, Moderna) covid vaccines. The CDC's Vaccine Safety Datalink was utilized for this purpose.

- The incidence rate of GBS was 324 per million person-years in the 1 to 21 day period following Janssen's covid vaccine, significantly higher than the background rate. It was 13 per million person-years after mRNA vaccination.

- During the first 3 weeks post-vaccine, the rate ratio (RR) of confirmed GBS cases after Janssen versus mRNA vaccination was 20.56 ($p < .001$), with 15.5 excess GBS cases in the risk interval per million Janssen vaccine recipients.

- Nearly all patients with GBS after Janssen's vaccination had facial weakness or paralysis, plus weakness and decreased reflexes in the limbs.

- Analyses of GBS were confirmed by medical records and adjudication.

- The Food and Drug Administration subsequently added a warning about Guillain-Barré syndrome to the Janssen vaccine fact sheet.

146.

All covid vaccines cause mild, severe, and fatal neurological adverse reactions

"This review shows that the spectrum of neurological side effects of [covid vaccination] is broad, ranging in severity from mild to severe, and that the outcome ranges from full recovery to death."

Finsterer J. **Neurological Adverse Reactions to SARS-CoV-2 Vaccines.** *Clin Psychopharmacol Neurosci* 2023 May 30: 21(2): 222-39.

- The author summarizes the nature, frequency, and outcome of neurological adverse reactions associated with covid vaccination.

- Disorders of the central nervous system triggered by covid vaccination include cerebro-vascular conditions (i.e., venous thrombosis, ischemic stroke, intra-cerebral hemorrhage), inflammatory diseases (i.e., encephalitis, meningitis, demyelinating disorders, transverse myelitis), and epilepsy.

- Disorders of the peripheral nervous system triggered by adverse reactions to covid vaccination include Guillain-Barré syndrome (GBS), Turner syndrome, small fiber neuropathy, myasthenia, and other conditions.

- The most common neurological side effects after covid vaccination are facial palsy, intracerebral hemorrhage, venous thrombosis, and GBS.

- All brands of covid vaccines cause adverse reactions that can be mild, severe, or fatal. They occur after any dose, in both sexes, and with variable latency periods (time to onset of symptoms) after vaccination.

- Although side effects can affect any organ or tissue of the body, the most commonly affected organ is the central or peripheral nervous system.

147.

Covid vaccination causes
Guillain-Barré syndrome

"These data suggested a clear and plausible excess of Guillain-Barré syndrome cases occurring within 42 days after the first dose of AstraZeneca's COVID-19 vaccination."

Keh RYS, Scanlon S, et al. **COVID-19 vaccination and Guillain-Barré syndrome: analyses using the National Immunoglobulin Database.** *Brain* 2023 Feb 13; 146(2): 739-48.

- This study investigated the relationship between covid vaccination and Guillain-Barré syndrome (GBS) using data from a national health database in England and UK hospitals.

- The first dose of AstraZeneca's covid vaccine was associated with an estimated excess GBS risk of 5.8 cases per million doses.

148.

Oo WM, Giri P, deSouza A. **AstraZeneca COVID-19 vaccine and Guillain-Barré syndrome in Tasmania: a causal link?** *J Neuroimmunol* 2021 Nov 15; 360: 577719.

"Nearly all reported cases of post-COVID-19 vaccination inflammatory demyelinating polyneuropathy are linked to AstraZeneca vaccination, and a variant with bifacial weakness is the most reported form of Guillain-Barré syndrome globally."

149.

Alijanzadeh D, Soltani A, et al. **Clinical characteristics and prognosis of temporary miller fisher syndrome following COVID.19 vaccination: a systematic review of case studies.** *BMC Neurol* 2023 Sep 21; 23(1): 332.

"Miller-Fisher syndrome (MFS) is a variant of Guillain–Barré syndrome. MFS must be considered in a list of the differential diagnoses in patients with a history of recent COVID-19 vaccination."

150.

GBS and facial nerve palsy occur more often after DNA/vector-based versus mRNA-based covid vaccines

"Molecular mimicry is often the primary pathogenic mechanism for vaccine-associated Guillain-Barré syndrome. Specifically, the vaccine contains the same structure as gangliosides, and thus vaccinated individuals produce anti-ganglioside antibodies that attack neural autoantigens, thereby causing neurological damage and associated clinical symptoms."

Yu M, Nie S, et al. **Guillain-Barré syndrome following COVID-19 vaccines: a review of literature.** *Front Immunol* 2023 Feb 15; 14:1078197.

• Chinese researchers analyzed 60 cases of Guillain-Barré syndrome (GBS) that occurred after covid vaccination.

• The average time from covid vaccination to onset of GBS was twelve days; 90% of cases occurred after the first dose. Initial symptoms included limb weakness, parethesia, and bilateral facial nerve palsy.

• Bilateral facial nerve palsy and facial palsy with distal paresthesia were more common for DNA/vector-based vaccines (AstraZeneca, Johnson & Johnson) than for mRNA-based vaccination (Pfizer, Sinovac).

151.

Ogunjimi OB, Tsalamandris G, et al. **Guillain-Barré syndrome induced by vaccination against COVID-19: a systematic review and meta-analysis.** *Cureus* 2023 Apr 14; 15(4): e37578.

"The pooled prevalence of GBS after vaccination against COVID-19 has been established to be 8.1 per one million vaccinations."

• A systematic review of 71 scientific papers on GBS post-covid vaccination was conducted. Other forms of GBS, such as bilateral facial nerve palsy and Miller-Fisher syndrome were included. Most cases of GBS were associated with a vector-based covid vaccine.

152.

WHO data reveal that GBS and facial palsy occur more often after vector-based versus mRNA covid vaccines

"Adenovirus-vectored COVID-19 vaccines are associated with higher reporting rates of GBS compared with mRNA-based COVID-19 vaccines."

Atzenhoffer M, Auffret M, et al. **Guillain-Barré syndrome associated with COVID-19 vaccines: a perspective from spontaneous report data.** *Clin Drug Investig* 2022 Jul; 42(7): 581-92.

- French scientists accessed the World Health Organization's pharmacovigilance database, VigiBase, to compare the risk of Guillain-Barré Syndrome (GBS) associated with mRNA-based (Pfizer and Moderna) and adenovirus-vectored (AstraZeneca and Janssen) covid vaccines.

- There were 3466 cases of GBS associated with covid vaccination in Vigibase, of which 967 (27.9%) were excluded, mainly due to poor quality data from Australia, Brazil, the US, and the UK. A total of 2499 reports from 39 nations were included in the analysis.

- Reporting rates for GBS were 13.9 and 55.7 per one million person-years for mRNA and vectored covid vaccines, respectively. The reporting rate per million doses administered was 6.40 for vectored covid vaccines combined, and 9.84 for Johnson & Johnson's Janssen vaccine.

- The reporting rate of GBS per million doses given was highest in Germany and the US for the Janssen covid vaccine: 12.56 and 12.24, respectively.

- The observed-to-expected (OE) ratio of GBS for onset within 3 weeks after vectored covid vaccination was 4.87, 5.76, 6.48, and 7.22 for Germany, the US, Spain, and the Netherlands, respectively. In the US, the OE ratio was significantly elevated after mRNA-based covid vaccines.

- Facial paralysis, including Bell's palsy, occurred in 9.6% of patients and was more frequent after vectored versus mRNA covid vaccines ($p < 0.001$).

- Of 716 patients with a reported outcome, 21.4 % recovered and 4.9% died.

153.

Bell's palsy and Guillain-Barré syndrome occur after MRNA covid vaccination

"Peripheral nervous system adverse events, especially Bell's palsy, should be carefully observed after mRNA vaccination against COVID-19."

Lai YH, Chen HY, et al. **Peripheral nervous system adverse events after the administration of mRNA vaccines: a systematic review and meta-analysis of large-scale studies.** *Vaccines (Basel)* 2022 Dec 17; 10(12): 2174.

- This study assessed the risk of peripheral nervous system (PNS) adverse events after mRNA covid vaccination.

- A systematic review of 15 studies was conducted. Bell's palsy and Guillain–Barré syndrome (GBS) had sufficient data for analysis.

- Bell's palsy has an incidence rate of 60.7 per million persons after the first dose of mRNA vaccination and 50.6 per million persons after the second dose. Without information on the dose of mRNA vaccination, the incidence rate of post-vaccination Bell's palsy is 310.8 per million persons.

- Individuals who received an mRNA covid vaccine were significantly more likely than the unvaccinated group to develop Bell's palsy, and Bell's palsy was significantly more likely after Pfizer's mRNA covid vaccine than Moderna's (odds ratio, OR = 1.64).

- The incidence of Bell's palsy after Pfizer's or Moderna's mRNA vaccine was higher than in the unvaccinated group.

- The risk of GBS was significantly higher after Pfizer's mRNA covid vaccine than after Moderna's (OR = 2.85).

- If studies that were excluded from this analysis were included, PNS adverse events after mRNA vaccination would be much higher.

154.

mRNA covid vaccination significantly increases the risk of Bell's palsy

"This study suggests that [Pfizer's] mRNA COVID-19 vaccine might be associated with increased risk of Bell's palsy. The overall observed rate of Bell's palsy after vaccination was higher than the expected rates."

Shibli R, Barnett O, et al. **Association between vaccination with the BNT162b2 mRNA COVID-19 vaccine and Bell's palsy: a population-based study.** *Lancet Reg Health Eur.* 2021 Dec; 11: 100236.

- Scientists used Israel's largest healthcare provider's database to assess the association between Pfizer's mRNA covid vaccine and Bell's palsy (facial paralysis). They tabulated cases within 21 days after the first dose and 30 days after the second dose, and compared them to pre-vaccine expected cases.

- In the 16 and older age group, the risk of Bell's palsy within 21 days after the first vaccine dose is 50.9 cases per one million people vaccinated. Females 45-64 years old have a higher risk: 62 cases per million, and females 65 and older have the worst rate: 74.1 cases per million people vaccinated.

- The mRNA covid vaccine significantly increases the risk of Bell's palsy, and this association is most pronounced in older women after the first dose.

- In vaccinated patients with a previous history of Bell's palsy, the risk of Bell's palsy within 21 days after the first vaccine dose is 528.6 cases per million people vaccinated, and even higher within 30 days after the second dose: 759.5 cases per million people vaccinated.

155.

Sato K, Mano T, et al. **Facial nerve palsy following the administration of COVID-19 mRNA vaccines: analysis of a self-reporting database.** *Int J Infect Dis* 2021 Oct; 111: 310-12.

"Our results showed a statistically significant association between the administration of mRNA COVID-19 vaccines and the reporting of facial nerve palsy after vaccination."

156.

Covid vaccination significantly increases the risk of Bell's palsy

"Using different study designs, with different underlying assumptions, findings from this study consistently show a safety signal and overall increased risk of Bell's palsy after CoronaVac vaccination."

Wan EYF, Chui CSL, et al. **Bell's palsy following vaccination with mRNA (BNT162b2) and inactivated (CoronaVac) SARS-CoV-2 vaccines: a case series and nested case-control study.** *Lancet Infect Dis* 2022 Jan; 22(1): 64-72.

• Using Department of Health data in Hong Kong, scientists assessed the risk of Bell's palsy after mRNA (Pfizer) and CoronaVac (Sinovac) vaccination.

• The incidence of confirmed Bell's palsy was 669 per one million person-years after CoronaVac vaccination and 428 per million after Pfizer vaccination.

• CoronaVac-vaccinated people were more than twice as likely as unvaccinated people to develop Bell's palsy (adjusted odds ratio, aOR = 2.39). Males were nearly three times as likely (aOR = 2.89).

• When the diagnosis of Bell's palsy was longer than 14 days post-vaccination, Pfizer-vaccinated people were nearly four time more likely than unvaccinated people to develop Bell's palsy (aOR = 3.78).

157.

Albakri K, Khaity A, et al. **Bell's palsy and COVID-19 vaccines: a systematic review and meta-analysis.** *Vaccines (Basel)* 2023 Jan 20; 11(2): 236.

"Most of the patients (62.8%) experienced unilateral facial paralysis."

• The authors reviewed 52 studies on Bell's palsy after covid vaccination. The rate after covid vaccination was 25.3 per one million. Most cases occurred after the first dose of Pfizer, AstraZeneca, and Sputnik vaccines. The average time to symptom onset post-vaccination was 11.6 days.

Covid Vaccine and Menstrual Irregularities

Several studies show that women have increased menstrual bleeding, pain, and clots after covid vaccination. It was also associated with a 72% higher risk of longer menstrual cycles in the first six months after vaccination. They had earlier cycles, longer periods, and heavier bleeding after the first and second doses. Covid-vaccinated women were significantly more likely than unvaccinated women to have doctor-related diagnoses for "excessive, frequent and irregular menstruation" (*International Classification of Diseases,* ICD code N92), and "other abnormal uterine and vaginal bleeding" (ICD code N93).

Exactly how the covid vaccine causes menstrual abnormalities is unknown. Post-vaccine menstrual disturbances may be related to an immunological/ inflammatory reaction. Another possibility is that diffusion of the spike protein in female tissues via mRNA-based vaccination may interfere with the endocrine homeostasis of the menstrual cycle. One study speculated that it may be from immune-mediated vaccine-induced thrombocytopenia. Another study found that menstrual changes were not caused by health-related behavioral factors or pandemic-related stress.

158.

Unusual menstrual bleeding patterns occur after covid vaccination

"We have documented a phenotype of increased menstrual bleeding after COVID-19 vaccination across a diverse set of currently and formerly menstruating people."

Lee KM, Junkins EJ, et al. **Investigating trends in those who experience menstrual bleeding changes after SARS-CoV-2 vaccination.** *Sci Adv* 2022 July 15; 8(28): eabm7201.

- Shortly after covid vaccines became available, many women reported that they experienced unexpected menstrual bleeding post vaccination. With no data to support these claims, their concerns were dismissed by health experts.

- This study surveyed 39,129 women between 18 and 80 years old to investigate menstrual bleeding patterns after covid vaccination among menstruating and non-menstruating women. All study participants were fully vaccinated and had not contracted covid.

- In this study, 42% of women with regular menstrual cycles bled more heavily than usual and 66% of post-menopausal women reported breakthrough bleeding after covid vaccination.

- Heavier menstrual flows after covid vaccination were more likely in women who were older, Hispanic, or had been pregnant in the past.

- The authors suggest that covid vaccination is more likely to be affecting menstrual bleeding patterns via inflammatory pathways rather than by ovarian hormone processes.

- The covid vaccination campaign might have revealed a poorly recognized side effect of highly immunogenic vaccines administered to women: systemic inflammatory responses that invoke downstream responses in target organs such as the uterus.

159.

Women have increased menstrual bleeding, pain, and clots after covid vaccination

"A major finding of this study is that almost 78% of the women surveyed reported changes in their menstrual cycle. The most frequent menstrual changes were: more menstrual bleeding and pain, delayed menstrual cycle, fewer days of menstrual bleeding, shorter cycle length, increased need for medication, and more or larger clots."

Baena-García L, Aparicio VA, et al. **Premenstrual and menstrual changes reported after COVID-19 vaccination: The EVA project.** *Womens Health (Lond)* 2022 Jan-Dec; 18: 17455057221112237.

- Although the menstrual cycle is an important physiological process for female health, it is poorly represented in scientific research. None of the clinical trials for covid vaccines considered health effects specific to women, such as menstrual disorders.

- After the covid vaccination campaign was initiated, many women reported that their premenstrual and menstrual patterns had changed.

- This study surveyed 14,153 women between 18 and 55 years of age to determine the prevalence of reported premenstrual and menstrual changes after covid vaccination.

- Of the women who participated in this study, 78% reported changes in their menstrual cycle post vaccination. They tended to be older ($p < 0.001$) and more likely to smoke ($p = 0.053$) than women who did not report any changes.

- Regarding premenstrual symptoms, the most prevalent changes post vaccination were increased fatigue, abdominal bloating, irritability, sadness, and headaches.

- The most prevalent menstrual changes post vaccination were increased menstrual bleeding (43%) and pain (41%), delayed menstruation (38%), fewer days of menstrual bleeding (35%), a shorter cycle (32%), increased need for medication (32%), and more or larger clots (29%).

160.

The covid vaccine is associated with menstrual changes and irregular bleeding

"Our study shows relatively high rates of irregular bleeding and menstrual changes after receiving the SARS-CoV-2 mRNA BNT162b2 vaccine."

Lessans N, Rottenstreich A, et al. **The effect of BNT162b2 SARS-CoV-2 mRNA vaccine on menstrual cycle symptoms in healthy women.** *Int J Gynaecol Obstet* 2023 Jan; 160(1): 313-318.

- This study investigated menstrual patterns and changes in 219 women who monitored their menstruation through electronic calendars before and after receiving a covid vaccine.

- Of all study participants, 38% reported menstrual changes and 23% experienced irregular bleeding post vaccination.

- Women who experienced irregular bleeding were more likely to have previously given birth to one or more children when compared to women with no irregular bleeding. They were also significantly more likely to have had medical comorbidities ($p = 0.003$).

161.

Blix K, Laake I, et al. **Unexpected vaginal bleeding and COVID-19 vaccination in nonmenstruating women.** *Sci Adv* 2023 Sep 22; 9(38): eadg1391.

"By use of data from two large population-based cohorts, we have observed an increased risk of unexpected vaginal bleeding after COVID-19 vaccination in non-menstruating women across different stages of reproductive aging."

- A total of 21,925 women were investigated. In pre- and peri-menopausal women, vaginal bleeding increased fivefold (adjusted hazard ratio, HR = 4.9) within four weeks after covid vaccination, as compared to the pre-vaccine period. In post-menopausal women, vaginal bleeding increased threefold (HR = 2.9).

162.

Doctor visits for excessive menstruation and abnormal vaginal bleeding surged during the covid vaccination campaign

"About 97,000 [suspected adverse effect] reports concern COVID-19 vaccines; out of those, approximately 7,000 apply to suspected menstrual disturbance, foremost heavier or breakthrough bleeding."

Edelman A, Boniface ER, et al. **Association between menstrual cycle length and coronavirus disease 2019 (COVID-19) vaccination: a U.S. cohort.** *Obstetrics & Gynecology* 2022 Apr 1; 139(4): 481-89.

- Covid-vaccinated women were significantly more likely than unvaccinated women to have doctor-related diagnoses for "excessive, frequent and irregular menstruation" (*International Classification of Diseases,* ICD code N92), and "other abnormal uterine and vaginal bleeding" (ICD code N93).

163.

Muhaidat N, Alshrouf MA, et al. **Menstrual symptoms after COVID-19 vaccine: a cross-sectional investigation in the MENA region.** *Int J Womens Health* 2022 Mar 28; 14: 395-404.

"The study showed a possible link between the COVID-19 vaccine and menstrual abnormalities that have impacted quality of life."

- This study investigated the prevalence and impact of menstrual abnormalities after covid vaccination in Middle Eastern and North African females.

- Of 2269 females 14 to 54 years of age, 66% experienced menstrual abnormalities post vaccination; 56% reported that the menstrual abnormalities they experienced after vaccination significantly affected their quality of life.

- Exactly how the covid vaccine causes menstrual abnormalities is unknown, though it may be from immune-mediated vaccine-induced thrombocytopenia since other vaccines, including MMR and pertussis, have been linked to vaccine-induced thrombocytopenia causing menstrual irregularities.

164.

The covid vaccine, not a covid infection, is associated with significant menstrual changes

"COVID-19 vaccination, but not SARS-CoV-2 infection, was associated with 1.7-fold increased risk of a short-term (<6 months) increase in usual menstrual cycle length. These results underscore the importance of monitoring menstrual health in vaccine clinical trials. Future work should examine the potential biological mechanisms."

Wang S, Mortazavi J, et al. **A prospective study of the association between SARS-CoV-2 infection and COVID-19 vaccination with changes in usual menstrual cycle characteristics.** *Am J Obstet Gynecol* 2022 Nov; 227(5): 739.e1-739.e11.

- This study was conducted to systematically investigate any associations between covid infection and covid vaccination with menstrual changes.

- In this study of 3,858 women, menstrual cycle length and regularity were measured prior to the covid pandemic (baseline, from 2011-2016), during the pandemic (late 2021), and post covid vaccination. The median age of the women at baseline and follow-up was 33 and 42 years, respectively.

- Covid vaccination was associated with a 72% higher risk of longer menstrual cycles in the first 6 months after vaccination (OR = 1.72, 95% CI = 1.08-2.73). Covid infection was not associated with any changes in usual menstrual characteristics, including cycle length or regularity.

- The link between covid vaccination and increased menstrual cycle length was most prevalent in women whose cycles at baseline (pre-pandemic) were normally irregular (either less than 26 days long or greater than 32 days long).

- Menstrual changes post vaccination occurred with mRNA (Pfizer, Moderna) and adenovirus-vectored vaccines (Johnson & Johnson). No differences were distinguished between brands of mRNA vaccines.

- This study also found that menstrual changes were not caused by health-related behavioral factors or pandemic-related stress.

165.

The covid vaccine is associated with menstrual irregularities such as longer periods and excessive bleeding

"Our preliminary report highlights that approximately 50-60% of reproductive age women who received the first dose of COVID-19 vaccine had menstrual cycle irregularities, regardless of the type of vaccine administered. The occurrence of menstrual irregularities seems to be slightly higher (60-70%) after the second dose."

Laganà AS, Veronesi G, et al. **Evaluation of menstrual irregularities after COVID-19 vaccination: Results of the MECOVAC survey.** *Open Med (Wars)* 2022 Mar 9; 17(1): 475-484.

- This study investigated menstrual irregularities and abnormal uterine bleeding after the first and second doses of the covid vaccine.

- Of the 164 participants in this study, more than half had menstrual irregularities—such as earlier cycles, longer periods, and heavier bleeding— after the first and second doses. These irregularities persisted for more than 2 months in 45% of the cases.

- After receiving a covid vaccine, many women had menstrual cycles that started 1-5 days earlier than expected, or more than 10 days early, periods lasting more than 7 days, and heavier than usual menstrual flows.

- Menstrual irregularities seemed to be more prevalent after the second dose, suggesting a potential additive effect.

- The study authors did not find differences between mRNA vaccines (by Pfizer and Moderna) and recombinant vaccines (by AstraZeneca and Janssen). Menstrual irregularities occurred regardless of the vaccine type or phase of the menstrual cycle at the time of vaccine administration.

- Post-vaccine menstrual disturbances may be related to an immunological/ inflammatory reaction. Another possibility is that diffusion of the spike protein in female tissues via mRNA-based vaccination may interfere with the endocrine homeostasis of the menstrual cycle.

166.

Cases of shedding of the entire mucus lining of the uterus significantly increased after covid vaccines were introduced

"This survey study showed a surge in decidual cast shedding experiences after the distribution of the COVID-19 vaccines."

Parotto T, Thorp JA, et al. **COVID-19 and the surge in decidual cast shedding.** *G Med Sci* 2022 Apr 21; 3(1): 107-117.

- This study provides evidence of a large increase in decidual cast shedding (DCS) after covid-19 vaccines were introduced. A decidual cast is when the entire thick mucus lining of the uterus sheds in one piece. Prior to the distribution of covid-19 vaccines, DCS was extremely rare.

- In this survey of 6,049 covid-19 vaccinated and unvaccinated women who were having menstrual irregularities, including many with severe symptoms, 292 women (4.83% of the sample) reported having experienced DCS.

- From April-June of 2021, after covid vaccines were widely utilized, google search terms for "decidual cast" increased by 2000% over prior months.

- The time frames for rapid increases in cases of DCS and google search terms for "decidual cast" and "decidual cast covid vaccine" align with the onset of widespread covid-19 vaccination.

- The rapid increase in DCS calls into question whether exposure to the spike protein, either naturally, from covid-19 vaccination, or from shedding of the spike protein through exosomes, is a factor.

- The authors hypothesize that a surge in menstrual abnormalities, including DCS, may be due to covid vaccines disrupting the hypothalamic-pituitary-ovarian axis. Also, nanolipid particles and "mRNA cargo" concentrate in the ovaries, producing an inflammatory response and bleeding disorders.

- The authors also speculate that DCS could be a tissue-like substance similar to fibrin-laden clots that morticians have discovered and removed post-mortem in some covid-vaccine recipients.

Additional Covid Vaccine Studies

Several studies show that serious adverse reactions are possible after covid vaccination. For example, Ajmera found that numerous vaccine recipients have died from gastrointestinal bleeding post-vaccination. Creutzfeldt-Jakob disease, a progressive neurodegenerative brain disorder, is also possible after covid vaccination. Hippisley-Cox found that having cancer, heart disease, or diabetes increases the risk of hospitalization or death after covid vaccination. Seneff provides evidence that mRNA covid vaccines cause innate immune suppression and may have cancer-causing properties. A team of South Korean scientists conducted two nationwide population-based studies and found that covid vaccines significantly increase the risk of autoimmune and psychiatric disorders.

Bardosh shows that Covid vaccine policies are harmful, unethical, scientifically unjustified, and a violation of human rights. In another study, it is shown that mandating covid vaccine booster shots for college students is unethical and causes more harm than benefit. Finally, Deruelle reviews pharmaceutical industry methods for manipulating information and science associated with the covid vaccine. He provides evidence that the pharmaceutical industry is dangerous to health and society, as revealed through industry tactics employed during the covid pandemic.

167.

Serious gastrointestinal adverse events such as diverticulitis and bowel perforation are possible after covid vaccination

"Vaccine recipients should be educated on vaccine-associated gastrointestinal adverse events in order to reduce morbidity and mortality. We also recommend that vaccine recipients with pre-existing GI disorders should be carefully monitored for the worsening of pre-existing conditions post-COVID-19 vaccination."

Ajmera K, Bansal R, et al. **Gastrointestinal complications of COVID-19 vaccines.** *Cureus* 2022 April 12; 14(4): e24070.

- This paper documented a case of acute diverticulitis and micro-perforation of the colon in a 41-year-old man following a booster dose of the Moderna covid vaccine. Additionally, the VAERS database was evaluated for gastrointestinal (GI) adverse events after covid vaccination.

- VAERS reports of GI-related adverse events that occurred after US covid vaccines were administered include diarrhea, abdominal pain, GI bleeding, diverticulitis, and bowel perforation.

- At least 100 vaccine recipients have died from GI bleeding post-vaccination while 431 patients with diarrhea post-vaccination have died. Thirteen of 36 patients (36.1%) with bowel perforation post-vaccination have died while 15 individuals with diverticulitis post-vaccination have died.

- Women 50-59 years of age had the highest incidence of GI-related adverse events following receipt of US covid vaccines produced by Pfizer, Moderna, and Janssen.

- Individuals with preexisting GI tract diseases, including those with a history of GI bleeding, inflammatory bowel disease, or peptic ulcers should be alerted to the risk of GI-related adverse events following covid vaccines.

- The authors hypothesize that the viral spike protein from the injected mRNA covid vaccine binds to cells in the GI tract promoting dysbiosis, inflammation, and other GI symptoms.

168.

Several cases of Creutzfeldt-Jakob disease, with symptoms manifesting shortly after covid vaccination, have been identified

"We present 26 cases of Creutzfeldt-Jakob disease, all diagnosed in 2021 with the first symptoms appearing within an average of 11.38 days after a Pfizer, Moderna, or AstraZeneca COVID-19 injection."

Perez, JC, Moret-Chalmin C, Montagnier L. **Emergence of a new Creutzfeldt-Jakob disease: 26 cases of the human version of mad cow disease, days after a COVID-19 injection.** *IJVTPR* 2023 Jan 12; 3(1): 727-770.

- Creutzfeldt-Jakob disease (CJD) is a fatal neurodegenerative brain disorder caused by prion proteins that have become pathogenic and transmissible. The authors document 26 cases of a rapidly developing prion disease. Twenty of the patients (77%) died within 5 months of vaccination.

- The senior author of this paper, Luc Montagnier, Nobel laureate, predicted the causation of this new form of CJD based on his genetic studies of pathogenic prion regions in the proteins of different species.

169.

Kuvandik A, Özcan E, et al. **Creutzfeldt-Jakob disease after the coronavirus disease-2019 vaccination.** *Turk J Intensive Care* 2022 Mar; 20(1): 61-64.

"In cases where rapidly progressive neurological disorders are observed, Creutzfeldt-Jakob disease should be considered."

- The authors present a case report of an elderly Turkish woman who developed neurological symptoms one day after her first dose of a covid-19 vaccine. She was admitted to the hospital with impaired vision, disorientation, regression, and inability to recognize the people around her.

- CJD is a contagious neurodegenerative disease with a 100% mortality rate. The patient died due to the rapid progression of the disease.

170.

mRNA covid vaccines cause innate immune suppression and may have cancer-causing properties

"Should any of these potentials be fully realized, the impact on billions of people around the world could be enormous and could contribute to both the short-term and long-term disease burden our health care system faces."

Seneff S, Nigh G, et al. **Innate immune suppression by SARS-CoV-2 mRNA vaccinations: The role of G-quadruplexes, exosomes, and MicroRNAs.** *Food Chem Toxicol* 2022 Jun; 164: 113008.

- This paper provides evidence that mRNA vaccines do not mimic a natural infection but instead suppress type I interferon responses that lead to impaired innate immunity. This leads to a cascading downstream effect that potentially causes increased infectious disease and cancer.

- The mRNA in the vaccine is hidden from cellular defenses. It produces an overabundance of the spike protein that diminishes DNA repair mechanisms.

- IFN-a and IRF9 play a central role in cancer surveillance and prevention. They are responsible for a fully functioning BRCA2 gene, which inhibits many types of cancer. IRF9 suppression via exosomal microRNA should be expected to impair the cancer-protective effects of BRCA2 gene activity.

- Vaccination has also been shown to suppress IRF7 and STAT2. This can interfere with the cancer-protective effects of BRCA1, which can lead to increased breast, uterine, ovarian, and pancreatic cancer in women. Men should see increased rates of prostate, breast, and pancreatic cancer.

- A review of the VAERS database found the following conditions: reactivation of varicella-zoster, immune thrombocytopenia, liver damage, Guillain Barré syndrome, Bell's palsy, demyelinating disease, hearing loss, myocarditis, cardiac failure, memory impairment, decreased mobility, and cognitive disorder.

- A search of mRNA covid vaccine in VAERS also found: cancer (breast, lung, prostate, colon), brain neoplasm, lymphoma, leukemia, and carcinoma.

171.

Covid vaccination causes an excess risk of serious adverse events

"These results raise concerns that mRNA vaccines are associated with more harm than initially estimated at the time of emergency authorization."

Fraiman J, Erveti J, et al. **Serious adverse events of special interest following mRNA COVID-19 vaccination in randomized trials in adults.** *Vaccine* 2022 Sept 22; 40(40): 5798-5805.

• This study investigated whether the Pfizer and Moderna covid vaccines were associated with an excess risk of serious adverse events. Pfizer had 101 "serious adverse events of special interest" per 100,000 vaccinated over placebo baselines. Moderna had an excess risk of 151 per 100,000 vaccinated.

• Some of the adverse events of special interest included acute respiratory distress, coagulation disorder, colitis/enteritis, myocarditis, other acute cardiac injury, and inflammation of the gall bladder.

172.

Hippisley-Cox J, Coupland CA, et al. **Risk prediction of covid-19 related death and hospital admission in adults after covid-19 vaccination: national prospective cohort study.** *BMJ* 2021 Sept 17; 374: n2244.

"This study...can be used to stratify risk populations to identify those who are at highest risk of severe covid-19 outcomes despite covid-19 vaccination."

• This study estimated the risk of covid-related mortality and hospital admission after covid vaccination, in people with various conditions. It considered more than 5 million adults 19-100 years of age who had received two doses.

• Hazard ratios were highest for patients with Down's syndrome (12.7-fold increase), kidney transplant (8.1), sickle cell disease (7.7), chemotherapy (4.3), home care residency (4.1), HIV/AIDS (3.3), liver cirrhosis (3.0), neurological conditions (2.6), dementia (2.2), and Parkinson's disease (2.2).

173.

Covid vaccination temporarily reduces sperm counts and converts into DNA inside human liver cells

"This longitudinal study demonstrates selective temporary sperm concentration and total motility count deterioration three months after [covid] vaccination, followed by later recovery."

Gat I, Kedem A, et al. **Covid-19 vaccination BNT162b2 temporarily impairs semen concentration and total motile count among semen donors.** *Andrology* 2022 Sep; 10(6): 1016-1022.

- This study analyzed 220 sperm samples from 37 sperm donors. Samples were compared before and after donors received two doses of the covid vaccine.

- Sperm concentration at 3 months post vaccination decreased by 15.4%, significantly lower ($p = 0.01$) compared to pre-vaccine measurements. The total motile count (the number of moving sperm in the entire ejaculate) also significantly declined at 3 months post vaccination, by 22.1% ($p = 0.007$).

174.

Aldén M, Falla FO, et al. **Intracellular reverse transcription of Pfizer BioNTech COVID-19 mRNA vaccine BNT162b2 in vitro in human liver cell line.** *Curr Issues Mol Biol* 2022 Feb 25; 44(3):1115-1126.

"We present evidence on fast entry of BNT162b2 [Pfizer's mRNA covid vaccine] into the [human liver] cells and subsequent intracellular reverse transcription of BNT162b2 mRNA into DNA."

- In petri dishes, researchers added Pfizer-BioNTech's mRNA covid vaccine to a human liver cell line. This study shows that the Pfizer covid vaccine enters human liver cells, induces changes in the LINE-1 gene and protein expression, and within 6 hours reverse transcription of the vaccine can be detected.

- This study did not investigate whether the converted DNA is integrated into the cells' DNA in the genome.

175.

mRNA covid vaccines significantly increase the risk of autoimmune and psychiatric adverse events

"Individuals in the mRNA vaccination cohort were at considerably higher risk of developing systemic lupus erythematosus (SLE) than those in the historical control cohort."

Jung S, Jeon JJ, et al. **Long-term risk of autoimmune diseases after mRNA-based SARS-CoV2 vaccination in a Korean, nationwide, population-based cohort study.** *Nat Commun* 2024 Jul 23; 15(1): 6181.

- South Korean scientists examined more that 9 million database records and determined that mRNA covid vaccines are significantly associated with systemic lupus erythematosus. Covid booster vaccines were also found to significantly increases the risk of alopecia, psoriasis, and rheumatoid arthritis.

- This study also found that women and patients over 40 years of age tended to a higher risk of bullous pemphigoid (an autoimmune blistering disease) after mRNA covid vaccination.

176.

Kim HJ, Kim N, et al. **Psychiatric adverse events following COVID-19 vaccination: a population-based cohort study in Seoul, South Korea.** *Mol Psychiatry* 2024 Jun 4; doi: 10.1038/s41380-024-02627-0.

"Our findings suggest that the relationship between covid vaccination and mental illness may be underestimated."

- South Korean scientists examined more than 2 million database records and determined that anxiety, dissociative disorders (e.g., memory loss or a blurred sense of identity), and somatoform disorders (e.g., social phobias or body dysmorphia), showed significantly increased risks after covid vaccination.

- Depression, sleep disorders, and sexual disorders also showed significantly higher cumulative incidence after covid vaccination.

177.

Informed consent forms for covid vaccine clinical trial subjects are inadequate, and rapid tests for diagnosing covid have variable accuracy

"Disclosure of the specific risk of worsened covid-19 disease from vaccination calls for a specific, separate, informed consent form and patient comprehension to meet medical ethics standards."

Cardozo T, Veazey R. **Informed consent disclosure to vaccine trial subjects of risk of COVID-19 vaccines worsening clinical disease.** *Int J Clin Pract* 2021 Mar; 75(3): e13795.

- This risk of antibody-dependent enhancement (ADE) with covid-19 vaccines was not adequately explained in clinical trial consent forms.

- The risk of ADE should have been "clearly and emphatically" described in disclosure forms and distinguished from rarely observed risks.

178.

Dinnes J, Deeks JJ, et al. **Rapid, point-of-care antigen and molecular-based tests for diagnosis of SARS-CoV-2 infection.** *Cochrane Database Syst Rev* 2021 Mar 24; 3(3): CD013705.

"Test accuracy studies cannot adequately assess the ability of antigen tests to differentiate those who are infectious and require isolation from those who pose no risk, as there is no standard for infectiousness."

- In this paper, 64 studies were reviewed to determine if rapid point-of-care (RPOC) tests, which can provide results in less than 2 hours, are accurate enough to diagnose covid infections.

- Tests varied in accuracy (from 58% to 95% in people with confirmed covid) depending on the different manufacturer brands and risk of bias in the analyzed studies. (Study bias included participant selection and weaknesses in the reference standard for ruling out a covid infection.)

179.

Covid-19 vaccine policies are harmful, unethical, scientifically unjustified, and a violation of human rights

"Mandatory vaccine policies are scientifically questionable and likely to cause more societal harm than good. Restricting people's access to work, education, public transport and social life based on COVID-19 vaccine status impinges on human rights, promotes stigma and social polarization, and adversely affects health and well-being."

Bardosh K, de Figueiredo A, et al. **The unintended consequences of COVID-19 vaccine policy: why mandates, passports and restrictions may cause more harm than good.** *BMJ Glob Health* 2022 May; 7(5): e008684.

- During the covid-19 pandemic, vaccine authorities enacted vaccine mandates, vaccine passports, and restrictions based on vaccination status. Evaluation of the unintended consequences of these policies has been limited.

- This paper describes why covid-19 vaccine policies may be harmful, assessing them from behavioral, political, legal, socioeconomic, and scientific outlooks.

- Covid vaccine policies appear to be non-evidence-based. They are punitive, discriminatory, and coercive, driven by factors that segregate, stigmatize, and polarize. The unvaccinated have been subjected to restrictive access to medical insurance and healthcare, fines, taxes, and threats of imprisonment.

- The media stifle debate by promoting simplistic narratives about alternate responses to the pandemic, and by labeling the unvaccinated as "anti-science."

- Vaccinated and unvaccinated people infect others at similar rates, and there is non-transparency regarding adverse effects such as blood clots.

- Covid vaccines were developed with public funds while pharmaceutical companies reap the profits but not the costs associated with adverse effects.

- Policies restricting the unvaccinated from work, education, public transportation and social life are violations of constitutional and human rights.

180.

Mandating covid-19 vaccine booster shots for college students is unethical and causes more harm than benefit

"Boosting young adults with [the Pfizer covid vaccine] could cause 18.5 times more serious adverse events per million (593.5) than COVID-19 hospitalizations averted (32.0). We urge universities and schools to rescind all COVID-19 vaccine mandates."

Bardosh K, Krug A, et al. **COVID-19 vaccine boosters for young adults: a risk benefit assessment and ethical analysis of mandate policies at universities.** *J Med Ethics* 2024 Jan 23; 50(2): 126-138.

- In 2021, an FDA advisory committee voted 16-2 against covid booster shots for healthy young adults but was overruled by the White House and CDC.

- In 2022, many US and Canadian colleges required their students to receive a third dose of the covid-19 vaccine. To assess the soundness of mandating covid-19 booster shots in young adults, the authors of this paper conducted a risk-benefit assessment and ethical analysis.

- More than 31,000 adults 18-29 years of age must receive a third covid vaccine to prevent one covid-related hospitalization during a 6-month period. Yet, for each covid hospitalization prevented, the vaccine is expected to cause at least 18 serious adverse events, including myopericarditis.

- For males 18-29 years of age who receive a covid booster shot, about 1 in 7000 (147 cases per million booster doses) will develop myocarditis within a few days. For males 16-17 years of age, the rate is 1 in 5000 (200 cases per million). The rate is 377 per million in males 12-17 years of age.

- Covid vaccine booster mandates to enroll (or remain) in college are unethical because they are not based on an updated risk-benefit assessment for college-age students, may cause more harm than good, are poorly effective against transmission, and vaccine injuries are not reliably compensated.

- Authorities who mandate covid vaccine boosters for young adults disregard the rapidly waning immunity, adverse effects, and benefits of prior infection.

181.

The pharmaceutical industry is dangerous to health and society, as revealed during the covid pandemic

"The unscientifically validated vaccination laws, originating from industry-controlled medical science, led to the adoption of social measures for the supposed protection of the public but which became serious threats to the health and freedoms of the population."

Deruelle F. **The pharmaceutical industry is dangerous to health. Further proof with COVID-19.** *Surg Neurol Int* 2022 Oct 21; 13(475): 1-18.

- The author reviews pharmaceutical industry methods for manipulating information and science associated with covid-19.

- Methods of information manipulation include, but are not limited to, falsified clinical trials, inaccessible data, fake or conflicted studies, concealment of vaccine side effects, banning alternative treatments, social engineering, behavior modification, and media censorship.

- Other manipulation strategies include funding journals to influence what is published, suppressing publication of unfavorable science, removing scientists from power, training people to be trusted voices for industry, and normalizing industry's presence in academic settings.

- Covid vaccines were tested in young and healthy populations rather than vulnerable elderly with comorbidities.

- The pharmaceutical industry invests in the media to control the dissemination of favorable information.

- Although huge profits are obtained by the pharmaceutical industry, the main goal appears to be mandatory vaccination with vaccine passports, consolidation of health data, and restriction of freedoms for the unvaccinated.

Covid and Vitamin D

The studies is this chapter provide strong evidence that vitamin D supplementation protects against severe covid morbidity and mortality. Individuals who are deficient in vitamin D are at increased risk of covid infection, hospitalization, and death. For example, in a study of ten European nations, researchers found that about 58% of the death rate from covid can be explained by the prevalence of severe vitamin D deficiency. Israeli scientists studied 7,807 people and found that low vitamin D levels significantly increased the risk of covid infection and hospitalization. Hosseini found that among hospitalized covid patients, admission into the intensive care unit (ICU) was related to a lower vitamin D level. Petrelli found that vitamin D supplementation reduced the risk of severe covid and covid death.

D'Avolio suggests taking 5,000 IU per day to reduce the risk of infection. The goal should be to raise the level to at least 40-60 ng/mL. People at risk of covid should consider taking 10,000 IU a day of vitamin D_3 for a few weeks to rapidly increase their concentrations. If you're unsure of your vitamin D status, you can take an at-home blood test that measures a form of the vitamin known as 25-hydroxyvitamin D, or request it from a healthcare practitioner.

182.

There is a significant association between severe vitamin D deficiency in European populations and the Covid-19 death rate

"There is a strong correlation between prevalence of severe vitamin D deficiency and the mortality rate per million from Covid-19 in European countries. Authors recommend for physicians to universally screen for vitamin D deficiency, and recommend further investigation of vitamin D supplementation in randomized control studies, which may lead to possible treatment or prevention of Covid-19."

Pugach IZ and Pugach S. **Strong correlation between prevalence of severe vitamin D deficiency and population mortality rate from Covid-19 in Europe.** *Wien Klin wochenschr* 2021 Apr; 133(7-8): 403-405.

- In the United States, blacks and Hispanics are known to have lower vitamin D levels than the general population, and these groups also have a higher mortality rate from Covid-19.

- In this study, researchers analyzed vitamin D population data from ten European nations to determine if vitamin D status is associated with the Covid-19 population death rate.

- A Pearson correlation analysis between prevalence of severe vitamin D deficiency and the Covid-19 death rate per million people showed a strong statistical relationship ($r = 0.76$, $p = 0.01$).

- Severe vitamin D deficiency is defined as a 25-hydroxyvitamin D level below 25 nmol/L (10 ng/mL).

- About 58% of the death rate from Covid-19 can be explained by the prevalence of severe vitamin D deficiency.

- The data shows a robust correlation between prevalence of severe vitamin D deficiency and Covid-19 deaths in ten European nations.

183.

A low plasma vitamin D level increases the risk of becoming infected and hospitalized with Covid-19

"We concluded that low plasma 25(OH)D levels appear to be an independent risk factor for COVID-19 infection and hospitalization."

Merzon E, Tworowski D, et al. **Low plasma 25(OH) vitamin D level is associated with increased risk of COVID-19 infection: an Israeli population-based study.** *FEBS J* 2020 Sep; 287(17): 3693-3702.

- Vitamin D deficiency has been recognized as a global pandemic. This study evaluated associations between plasma 25-hydroxyvitamin D levels with the likelihood of becoming infected and hospitalized with Covid-19.

- Israeli scientists measured vitamin D levels in 7,807 individuals, including 782 who were Covid-19-positive and 7,025 who were Covid-19-negative.

- A low plasma 25-hydroxyvitamin D level was found to significantly increase the risk of Covid-19 infection (OR = 1.58) and hospitalization (OR = 2.09).

- This study found that suboptimal plasma vitamin D levels increase the risk for Covid-19 infection and hospitalization, independent of pre-existing medical conditions and demographic characteristics.

184.

Israel A, Schäffer AA, et al. **Identification of drugs associated with reduced severity of COVID-19—a case-control study in a large population.** *Elife* 2021 Jul 27: 10:e68165.

- A large Israeli database of over 4.7 million health care records was used for this study seeking products that are protective against severe covid disease.

- Vitamin D was one of the products that significantly reduced the odds for covid hospitalization (OR = 0.87).

185.

Vitamin D deficiency increases covid disease incidence and severity

"Vitamin D supplementation may have prevention or treatment potential for COVID-19 disease."

Ye K, Tang F, et al. **Does serum vitamin D level affect COVID-19 infection and its severity? A case-control study.** *J Am Coll Nutr* 2021 Nov-Dec; 40(8); 724-31.

- The study evaluated the relationship between the vitamin D serum level and covid infection and severity. It compared 62 hospitalized covid patients and 80 healthy controls. Cases were categorized by severity.

- Vitamin D levels in severe covid cases (38.2 nmol/L or 15.3 ng/mL) were significantly lower than in mild/moderate cases (56.6 nmol/L or 22.7 ng/mL).

- Vitamin D deficiency was found in 41.9% of covid cases but in only 11.1% of healthy controls.

- There was a statistically significant association between vitamin D deficiency and severe/critical covid disease (odds ratio, OR = 15.18).

186.

Ranjbar M, Karbalaie Niya MH, et al. **Serum level of vitamin D is associated with COVID-19 mortality rate in hospitalized patients.** *J Res Med Sci* 2021 Nov 29; 26: 112.

"Our study showed that a lower level of serum level of Vitamin D is associated with a higher mortality rate in patients with COVID-19 independent of age and sex."

- Of 317 hospitalized covid patients, admission into the intensive care unit was related to a lower vitamin D level (odds ratio, OR = 8.57, $p < 0.001$).

- A significant association was found between high levels of serum vitamin D and protection against death.

187.

Covid patients have significantly lower vitamin D levels

"It is probable that vitamin D_3 supplementation would be useful in the treatment of COVID-19 infection, in preventing a more severe symptomatology and/or in reducing the presence of the virus in the upper respiratory tract and making the patients less infectious."

D'Avolio A, Avataneo V, et al. **25-Hydroxyvitamin D concentrations are lower in patients with positive PCR for SARS-CoV-2.** *Nutrients* 2020 May 9; 12(5): 1359.

• Statistically significantly lower vitamin D levels ($p = 0.004$) were found in people who tested positive for covid (median value 11.1 ng/mL) compared with those who tested negative (24.6 ng/mL).

• People at risk of covid should consider taking 10,000 IU a day of vitamin D_3 for a few weeks to rapidly increase their concentrations, then switch to 5,000 IU a day to reduce the risk of infection. The goal should be to raise the level to at least 40-60 ng/mL.

188.

Cozier YC, Castro-Webb N, et al. **Lower serum 25(OH)D levels associated with higher risk of COVID-19 infection in U.S. Black women.** *PLoS ONE* 2021 Jul 27; 16(7): e0255132.

"The present results suggest that U.S. Black women with lower levels of 25(OH)D are at increased risk of infection with COVID-19."

• Black people commonly experience vitamin D insufficiency (20 to 29 mg/mL) or deficiency (< 20 ng/mL) because darker skin pigmentation produces less vitamin D_3 when exposed to sunlight.

• A total or 1,974 Black women were included in this study. Compared to women with sufficient vitamin D levels (30 ng/mL or higher) women with insufficient or deficient amounts were significantly more likely to contract covid (age-adjusted OR = 1.44 and 1.73, respectively).

189.

Vitamin D has beneficial effects that protect against covid

"Data of the present study shed a brighter light on the still partially unresolved issue about vitamin D beneficial effects observed in patients with IL-6-related inflammation such as COVID-19 infection, suggesting a possible molecular mechanism by which this vitamin exerts its action."

Cimmino G, Conte S, et al. **Vitamin D inhibits IL-6 pro-atherothrombotic effects in human endothelial cells: a potential mechanism for protection against COVID-19 infection?** *J Cardiovasc Dev Dis* 2022 Jan 13; 9(1): 27.

- The authors studied the effect of vitamin D on Tissue Factor and cell adhesion molecules (CAMs) in IL-6-stimulated endothelial cells. ACE2r gene and proteins, and the modulation of NF-kB and STAT3 pathways, were also studied.

- Vitamin D significantly decreased Tissue Factor expression at gene and protein levels, and Tissue Factor-procoagulant functioning in IL-6-treated HUVEC. Similar effects occurred for CAMs and ACE2r expression.

- IL-6 precipitates endothelial dysfunction with Tissue Factor and CAMs expression via upregulation of ACE2r. Vitamin D impedes these IL-6 harmful effects so this may be how its beneficial effects in covid infection occur.

190.

Meltzer DO, Best TJ, et al. **Association of vitamin D status and other clinical characteristics with COVID-19 test results.** *JAMA Netw Open* 2020 Sep 3; 3(9): e2019722.

"These findings appear to support vitamin D status in Covid-19 risk. The low costs of vitamin D and it's general safety at doses of up to 4000 IU per day, support population-level supplementation."

- Subjects who tested positive for Covid-19 were significantly more likely to have been categorized as "likely deficient" (< 20 ng/mL) in vitamin D status as compared to those who were "likely sufficient" (relative risk, RR = 1.77).

191.

Vitamin D protects against
the most severe covid infections

"SARS-CoV-2 positivity is strongly and inversely associated with circulating 25(OH)D levels, a relationship that persists across latitudes, races/ethnicities, both sexes, and age ranges."

Kaufman HW, Niles JK. **SARS-CoV-2 positivity rates associated with circulating 25-hydroxyvitamin D levels.** *PloS ONE* 2020 Sep 17; 15(9): e0239252.

- This study was designed to determine if there is an association between vitamin D and severe acute covid infection.

- Out of 32,190 patients with deficient 25-hydroxyvitamin D levels (< 20 ng/mL) 12.5% were positive for severe acute covid infection, while only 8.1 % of 27,870 patients with adequate values (30-34 ng/mL) tested positive.

- Out of 12,321 patients with vitamin D values ≥ 55 ng/mL just 5.9% tested positive for severe acute covid infection.

- Regression analysis showed a strong correlation ($r^2 = 0.96$) between lower vitamin D levels and covid positivity in the total population.

192.

Hosseini B, El Abd A, Ducharme FM. **Effects of vitamin D supplementation on COVID-19 related outcomes: a systematic review and meta-analysis.** *Nutrients* 2022 May 20; 14(10): 2134.

"Our findings suggest that vitamin D supplementation, administered in hospitalized COVID-19 patients, is associated with a significant reduction in mortality, intensive care unit (ICU) admission, and need for mechanical ventilation."

- This systematic review and meta-analysis affirmed that vitamin D supplementation significantly reduced the risk of admission to an intensive care unit due to covid (RR = 0.35) and reduced covid mortality (RR = 0.46).

193.

Vitamin D is protective against covid infection, severity, and death

"Reduced vitamin D values resulted in a higher infection risk, mortality and severity of COVID-19 infection. Supplementation may be considered as a preventive and therapeutic measure."

Petrelli F, Luciani A, et al. **Therapeutic and prognostic role of vitamin D for COVID-19 infection: a systematic review and meta-analysis of 43 observational studies.** *J Steroid Biochem Mol Biol* 2021 Jul; 211: 105883.

- In this meta-analysis on the relationship between vitamin D levels and covid infection, 43 studies were considered. Those who were deficient in vitamin D (<20 ng/mL) were 50% more likely than non-deficient subjects to develop covid infection (odds ratio, OR = 1.5; p = .02).

- Vitamin D deficiency was also associated with more severe disease (OR = 2.6; p < .01) and higher mortality (OR = 1.22; p < .01).

- Vitamin D supplementation reduced the risk of severe covid (OR = 0.27; p < .01) and covid death (OR = 0.41; p = .01).

194.

Bayrak H, Öztürk D, et al. **Association between vitamin D levels and COVID-19 infection in children: a case-control study.** *Turk Arch Pediatr* 2023 May; 58(3): 250-255.

"Children with COVID-19 have a lower 25(OH)-D vitamin level compared to the control group."

- This study compared the vitamin D levels of 73 hospitalized pediatric covid patients to 76 healthy controls.

- The mean 25(OH)-D level in covid patients was 15.80 ng/mL and 21.51 ng/mL in the controls. The vitamin D level was statistically significantly lower in the covid patients compared to the healthy controls (p < .001).

Face Masks

Several studies show that face masks are ineffective at preventing the spread of covid. Additionally, when encountering mask-wearers, people reduce the space between them, increasing the risk of covid transmission. A systematic review of face masks reveals that they cause several side effects and safety issues. They may cause toxic levels of carbon dioxide and contain potentially risky chemical substances. Face masks also pollute the environment and are a threat to aquatic ecosystems. Plus, they inhibit people from recognizing facial expressions and impair the accuracy of interpreting emotional expression.

195.

A systematic review of face masks reveals several side effects and safety issues

"The policy of mandatory mask wearing was established by assuming that the population was a potential vector of infection and that the use of face masks was free from side effects."

Balestracci B, La Regina M, et al. **Patient safety implications of wearing a face mask for prevention in the era of COVID-19 pandemic: a systematic review and consensus recommendations.** *Intern Emerg Med* 2023 Jan; 18(1): 275-96.

- Due to the covid pandemic, wearing a face mask has been recommended.

- To investigate potential side effects and safety issues associated with wearing a face mask, the authors conducted a systematic review of 63 eligible papers published between 1995 and January 2022.

- Side effects and safety issues include breathing difficulties, dry eye and inflammation, skin reactions, anxiety and panic attacks. Also, communication and concentration problems, reduced working capacity, respiratory difficulties, fogging glasses, and headaches.

- Face masks may increase breathing resistance, decrease oxygen content, increase carbon dioxide, humidity, temperature, and pressure on the face, head, neck, nose and ears. Face masks may induce a sense of suffocating, worsening mood, depressive symptoms, and hyperventilation which can cause seizures.

- Face masks decrease the quality of life and can cause increased face touching and spread of covid. They also create a false sense of security resulting in reduced compliance with other measures.

- Wearing a N95 respirator is associated with worse side effects than wearing a cloth or surgical mask.

- People with breathing difficulties, young children and unconscious people may be contraindicated. Children with autism struggle to tolerate face masks.

196.

Mandatory face masks cause clinically relevant adverse health effects

"In the case of viral infections, masks appear to be not only less effective than expected, but also not free of undesirable biological, chemical, physical and psychological side effects."

Kisielinski K, Giboni P, et al. **Is a mask that covers the mouth and nose free from undesirable side effects in everyday use and free of potential hazards?** *Int J Environ Res Public Health* 2021 Apr 20; 18(8): 4344.

- Although many countries required masks to control the spread of covid-19, the adverse health effects of wearing masks were never fully investigated.

- The World Health Organization originally did not recommend widespread use of masks due to the dangers of self-contamination, breathing difficulties, a false sense of security, and potential adverse effects.

- In this paper, researchers evaluated 65 studies that scientifically confirmed numerous physical and psychological side effects of extended mask use.

- Masks have numerous statistically significant adverse health effects, including increased blood carbon dioxide, decreased blood oxygen saturation and cardio-pulmonary capacity, increased blood pressure, increased respiratory and heart rates, fatigue, exhaustion, headache, dizziness, and facial skin lesions.

- This paper showed a statistically significant link between mask-induced hypoxia and fatigue ($p < 0.05$). Both healthy and sick people can experience Mask-Induced Exhaustion Syndrome (MIES).

- Mask wearers exhale smaller particles than maskless people and their louder speech magnifies this increased production of fine aerosol particles.

- Studies suggest that mask use does not impact covid-19 infections. Infected versus uninfected groups of people did not differ in their use of masks.

- During the covid pandemic, the mask provided symbolic, psychological support for the general population to reduce anxiety in the community.

197.

Face masks do not prevent covid or other respiratory illnesses

"Wearing masks in the community probably makes little or no difference to the outcome of laboratory-confirmed influenza/SARS-CoV-2 compared to not wearing masks."

Jefferson T, Dooley L, et al. **Physical interventions to interrupt or reduce the spread of respiratory viruses.** *Cochrane Database Syst Rev* 2023 Jan 30; 1(1): CD006207.

- The authors of this paper identified 78 relevant studies, including 11 new randomized controlled studies (with 610,000 participants) from the covid-19 pandemic, to evaluate the effectiveness of physical interventions to interrupt or reduce the spread of respiratory viruses.

- The studies were conducted in various settings, ranging from schools and hospitals in high-income nations to inner cities in low-income nations.

- Medical/surgical masks were compared to not wearing masks. No statistical differences were found in the prevention of influenza-like illness or covid.

- The authors also found that the use of N95/P2 respirators compared to medical/surgical masks appeared to make little or no difference regarding laboratory-confirmed influenza.

- Hand-washing showed a 14% relative reduction in the number of people with acute respiratory infections.

- Potential harms associated with physical interventions were insufficiently investigated in the studies.

198.

When encountering mask-wearers, people reduce the space between them, increasing the risk of covid transmission

"Our finding implied that not only masks, but also vaccination could lead to the shortening of interpersonal distance and may cause challenges in the prevention and control of COVID-19 transmission."

Chen YL, Rahman A. **Effects of target variables on interpersonal distance perception for young Taiwanese during the COVID-19 pandemic.** *Healthcare (Basel)* 2023 June 11; 11(12): 1711.

- The authors surveyed 50 male and 50 female participants to investigate the effects of mask wearing and vaccination on interpersonal distance.

- Shorter distances were reported when participants encountered mask wearers versus non-mask wearers: 4 feet, 9 inches vs. 6 feet, 5 inches. Similar distances were reported when encountering vaccinated versus unvaccinated individuals.

- Interpersonal distances were just three feet when encountering masked *and* vaccinated individuals.

199.

Yan Y, Bayham J, et al. **Risk compensation and face mask mandates during the COVID-19 pandemic.** *Sci Rep* 2021 Feb 4; 11(1): 3174.

"Masks are associated with risk compensation behavior and Americans spend less time at home when living with a face mask mandate."

- The authors compared time that individuals spent at home versus visiting public locations that could more readily expose them to covid transmission, before and after face mask mandates were instituted.

- Americans subject to mask mandates spend 10-24 fewer minutes at home, increasing visits to commercial locations such as restaurants, which are high-risk for viral transmission. Thus, mask mandates could increase covid cases.

200.

Masked and quarantined military recruits contracted and spread covid

"Our study showed that in a group of predominantly young male military recruits, approximately 2% became positive for SARS-CoV-2... during a 2-week, strictly enforced quarantine."

Letizia AG, Ramos I, et al. **SARS-CoV-2 Transmission among Marine recruits during quarantine.** *NEJM* 2020 Dec 17; 383(25): 2407-16.

- This study investigated covid infections among 1848 Marine recruits who had quarantined for two weeks at home and then again for two weeks upon admission to basic training.

- All recruits and supervisors wore double-layered cloth masks at all times, except when sleeping or eating, and practiced social distancing.

- Of the 1801 recruits who had negative covid tests at enrollment, 35 (1.9%) tested positive on day 7 or day 14, despite a rigorous mask requirement and a strictly enforced quarantine.

201.

Hakre S, Malijkovic-Berry I, et al. **Transmission of SARS-CoV-2 among recruits in a US Army training environment: a brief report.** *J Public Health (Oxf)* 2023 Aug 28; 45(3): 748-52.

"Measures, such as masking and social distancing, were maintained throughout quarantine and basic combat training."

- Among 1403 US Army recruits, despite masking and social distancing, three covid transmission clusters occurred during quarantine.

- By the end of basic training, 1.5% of masked and previously quarantined military trainees developed covid. This occurred prior to the emergence of more transmissible strains.

- This report was sponsored by the US Department of Defense.

202.

Mask mandates do not reduce covid cases

"Results suggest that while it imposes a burden on the public, the use of face masks outdoors is not correlated with a decrease in the number of COVID-19 cases."

Alfano V, Cicatiello L, Ercolano S. **Assessing the effectiveness of mandatory outdoor mask policy: the natural experiment of Campania.** *Econ Hum Biol* 2023 Aug; 50: 101265.

- The authors compared the growth of covid cases in one region of Italy, Campania, that enforced the use of face masks outdoors, to the other Italian provinces that had no such mandate. A mask mandate did not reduce covid cases.

203.

Beauchamp JD, Mayhew CA. **Revisiting the rationale of mandatory masking.** *J Breath Res* 2023 Aug 7; 17(4):

"There is no statistically significant or unambiguous scientific evidence to justify mandatory masking for general, healthy populations with the intention of lessening the viral spread."

- There is no clear scientific proof that masks reduce covid transmission, so mandatory masks are unjustifiable and must be rejected in future policies.

204.

Juutinen A, Sarvikivi E, et al. **Face mask recommendations in schools did not impact COVID-19 incidence among 10-12 year-olds in Finland — joinpoint regression analysis.** *BMC Pub Health* 2023 Apr 21; 23(1): 730.

"Face mask recommendations in schools did not reduce COVID-19 incidence among 10–12 year-olds in Finland."

- This study compared covid incidence among 10-12 year-olds in cities with different face mask recommendations. Masks did not reduce covid.

205.

Inhaled air in masks could expose people to dangerous levels of carbon dioxide

"In view of the possible toxicological mask effects of re-breathed carbon dioxide in pregnant women, children and adolescents, and in view of the limited scientific evidence for masks as an effective pandemic measure, there is a need to re-evaluate and reconsider mask mandates especially for these vulnerable subgroups."

Kisielinski K, Wagner S, et al. **Possible toxicity of chronic carbon dioxide exposure associated with face mask use, particularly in pregnant women, children and adolescents – a scoping review.** *Heliyon* 2023 Apr; 9(4): e14117.

- The authors reviewed 43 scientific papers to investigate the toxicological effects of re-breathing carbon dioxide (CO_2) while wearing a face mask, specifically regarding pregnant women, children, and adolescents.

- Mask use can lead to carbon dioxide levels exceeding the National Institute for Occupational Safety and Health (NIOSH) and European exposure limits, both acutely and chronically.

- Fresh air has about 0.04% CO_2 while studies indicate that wearing a mask for more than five minutes exposes humans to 1.41%-3.2% CO_2, 35-80 times higher than normal.

- Depending on exposure time (from 1 to 60 minutes), CO_2 concentrations in the inhaled air under masks can range from 0.42% to 3.52%.

- Animal studies show that CO_2 levels above 0.3%, 0.5%, and 0.8% of inhaled air can lead to neuron damage, impaired learning, fetal death, and birth defects.

- There could be a developmental risk to early life and healthy children from prolonged mask wearing.

- Of 16 randomized controlled trials evaluating the efficacy of masks, just two (12.5%) showed a statistically significant benefit.

206.

Masks may cause toxic levels of carbon dioxide (CO_2) and contain potentially risky chemical substances

"The use of masks increased the CO_2 concentration in the air behind them to levels historically associated with toxicity."

Akhondi H, Kaveh S, et al. **CO_2 levels behind and in front of different protective mask types.** *HCA Healthc J Med* 2022 Aug 29; 3(4): 231-37.

- This study measured carbon dioxide (CO_2) levels behind and in front of face masks during continuous use.

- There were significantly higher CO_2 concentrations behind the mask compared to the front within an average of less than one hour of continuous use.

- Of all subjects, 77% had a behind-the-mask CO_2 concentration of more than 2000 ppm (the threshold for symptoms), while 12% had at least 5000 ppm (occupational health exposure limit).

- Younger age, warm ambient temperature, an N-95 mask, and exercise were most conducive to inducing extremely high CO_2 levels that should be avoided.

207.

Guo Y, Liu Y, et al. **Disposable polypropylene face masks: a potential source of micro/nanoparticles and organic contaminates in humans.** *Environ Sci Technol* 2023 Apr 11; 57(14): 5739-50.

"This study highlights the need to study the long-term health risks associated with mask wearing and raises concerns over mask quality control."

- The authors measured micro/nanoparticles and organic chemicals in disposable face masks. They found 79 semi-volatile organic compounds in masks, of which 18 were detected in at least 80% of samples.

- There is a risk of chemical exposure via particle inhalation.

208.

Face masks release high amounts of toxic chemicals

"Dimethylformamide (DMF) and dimethylacetamide (DMAc), which are organic solvents used in the production of masks, cause reproductive toxicity, liver toxicity, and cancer in the human body."

Ryu H, Kim Y. **Measuring the quantity of harmful volatile organic compounds inhaled through masks.** *Eco Toxicol Environ Saf* 2023 May; 256: 114915.

- The covid-19 pandemic established a global norm of mandatory mask wearing.

- In this study, scientists measured the concentration of volatile organic compounds (VOCs) emitted from commonly used masks.

- In KF94 masks, 1-methoxy-2-propanol, *N,N*-dimethylacetamide, n-hexane, and 2-butanone were detected at concentrations 22 to 147 times greater than those found in cotton masks.

- In some KF94 masks, the total VOCs released reached over 4000 μg m^{-3}, a risk to human health.

- Mask temperature may increase due to body heat. When the mask temperature rises, concentrations of the VOCs emitted from the mask can increase as well.

- This study showed that KF94 disposable masks released higher concentrations of total VOCs than cotton masks, high enough to pose a concern.

- Exposure to the highest concentrations of VOCs can be reduced if a mask is opened and unused for at least 30 minutes.

209.

Face masks are polluting the environment and are a threat to marine wildlife

"The improper disposal of personal protective equipment [face masks] used to protect against the spread of SARS-CoV-2 has aggravated the problem of marine plastic pollution."

Karthikeyan P, Subagunasekar M, et al. **Abundance, spatial distribution, and chemical characterization of face masks on the beaches of SE Kanyakumari, India.** *Mar Pollut Bull* 2023 Jul; 192: 115031.

- This study provides data on face mask pollution and highlights the need to optimize disposal of face masks.

- The study area consisted of 11 beaches in India polluted with face masks. A total of 1593 face masks were collected and assessed for abundance, spatial distribution, and chemical analysis.

- Birds, mammals, and invertebrates have been entangled in littered face masks. Masks have also been consumed by marine wildlife.

- Face masks are a new and important source of single-use plastics that are polluting the environment and causing a problem for ecosystems. Long-term management of waste face masks is required.

210.

Merad Y, Belmokhtar Z, et al. **Fungal contamination of medical masks among forensic healthcare workers in the COVID19 era.** *New Microbes New Infect* 2023 Apr 26; 53: 101134.

"The current study found that the high fungal contamination on the inside of the used surgical masks was most likely related to mask-wearing duration, environmental contamination, or healthcare worker's habits."

- In this study of 52 used masks collected from healthcare workers, 25 (48%) tested positive for fungal contamination. Alternaria, Penicillium, and Aspergillus were the most common fungi detected on the inside areas of the masks.

211.

Micro-fibers from used masks threaten aquatic ecosystems

"Inappropriate disposal of used surgical face masks...is the major cause of micro-fiber pollution."

Priya KK, Thilagam H, et al. **Impact of microfiber pollution on aquatic biota: a critical analysis of effects and preventive measures.** *Sci Total Environ* 2023 Aug 20; 887: 163984.

- Random disposal of used face masks end up in waterways. Face masks made of polymer materials release micro-plastics and fibers into the environment. Plankton in the food chain of the marine ecosystem are detrimentally impacted by micro-fibers.

212.

Jiang A, Pei W, et al. **Toxic effects of aging mask microplastics on E. coli and dynamic changes in extracellular polymeric matter.** *Sci Total Environ* 2023 Nov 15; 899: 165607.

"This study proposed the possible toxicity mechanism of mask microplastics...and provided a reference for future research on the toxic effects of mask microplastics on environmental organisms."

213.

Khoironi A, Hadiyanto H, et al. **Impact of disposable mask microplastics pollution on the aquatic environment and microalgae growth.** *Environ Sci Pollut Res Int* 2023 Jul; 30(31): 77453-68.

"The improper management of disposable mask waste has led to the increase of marine pollution, in terms of water quality, and the decline in aquatic microorganisms."

- Scientists investigated the affect of disposable mask waste on fresh water and microalgae biomass quality. Disposable masks decreased water quality and damaged microalgae by inhibiting their growth.

214.

Masks contain contaminants that could adversely affect human health

"Face mask-wearing as a public health measure to contain the spread of COVID-19 could be a potential risk factor for human health."

Tesfaldet YT, Ndeh NT. **Public face masks wearing during the COVID-19 pandemic: a comprehensive analysis is needed for potential implications.** *J Hazard Mater Adv* 2022 Aug; 7: 100125.

- This paper discusses benefits and risks of wearing face masks and recommends areas for additional research.

- Studies reveal that masks release micro-plastics and other contaminants such as endocrine disrupting ultraviolet stabilizers, nanofiber-infused nanoparticles, heavy metals and dyes, that could have an adverse effect on humans.

- Naphthalene, listed as a possible human carcinogen by the US Environmental Protection Agency, was detected in masks collected from several nations.

- The effects of temperature, moisture, humidity, and breathing rate on mask wearing should be investigated in greater detail.

215.

Jin L, Griffith SM, et al. **On the flip side of mask wearing: increased exposure to volatile organic compounds and a risk-reducing solution.** *Environ Sci Technol* 2021 Oct 19; 55(20): 14095-14104.

"Hazardous chemicals in the petroleum-derived polymer layer of masks are currently ignored and unregulated. These organic compounds pose potential health risks to the mask wearer through dermal contact or inhalation."

- The authors show that masks from around the world contain volatile organic compounds, including alkanes, polycyclic aromatic hydrocarbons, phthalate esters, and reactive carbonyls.

216.

Masks inhibit people from recognizing facial expressions

"The accuracy of emotion recognition in children was impaired for various facial expressions (disgust, fear, happy, neutral, sad, and surprise faces), except for angry faces."

Miyazaki Y, Kamatani M, et al. **Effects of wearing an opaque or transparent face mask on the perception of facial expressions: a comparative study between Japanese school-aged children and adults.** *Perception* 2023 Nov; 52(11-12): 782-798.

- This study assessed the ability of school-aged children to read the emotions of adults wearing face masks.

- Children were more impaired than adults at reading facial expressions hidden by face masks.

217.

Thomas, PJN, Caharel S. **Do masks cover more than just a face? A study on how facemasks affect the perception of emotional expressions according to their degree of intensity.** *Perception* 2024 Jan; 53(1): 3-16.

"Our results revealed a strong impact of facemasks on the recognition of expressions of disgust, happiness, and sadness, resulting in a decrease in performance and an increase in misinterpretations. In contrast, the recognition of anger and fear, as well as neutral expression, was found to be less impacted by mask-wearing."

- This study evaluated the impact that face masks have on interpreting emotional expressions.

- Wearing face masks during the covid pandemic has disrupted the human ability to decipher emotions from faces.

Obesity

About 3 billion people (39% of the global population) are obese. More than half of the population is expected to be obese by 2035. Obesity is defined as a body mass index (a measure of body fat based on height and weight) of ≥ 30.

Obesity increases the risk of many other diseases and health problems. In this chapter, several studies show that obesity significantly reduces influenza and covid vaccine efficacy. It also significantly increases the risk of developing a severe case of covid requiring hospitalization and intensive care. Nations with the highest proportions of overweight and obese adults have the worst covid death rates.

218.

Influenza vaccine efficacy is suboptimal in the obese population

"We report here, for the first time, that influenza vaccine antibody levels decline significantly and CD8⁺ T-cell responses are defective in obese compared with healthy weight individuals."

Sheridan PA, Paich HA, et al. **Obesity is associated with impaired immune response to influenza vaccination in humans.** *Int J Obes (Lond)* 2012 Aug; 36(8): 1072-77.

- Although more than two-thirds of the U.S. adult population is overweight or obese, humoral and cellular immune responses to influenza vaccination were never compared in healthy weight and overweight populations.

- This study measured antibody responses to the influenza vaccine in healthy weight, overweight and obese adults at 1 and 12 months post-vaccination. It also analyzed cellular immunity in influenza-stimulated cultures.

- At 1 month post-vaccination, a 10-unit increase in body mass index (BMI) increased antibody titer by 13%. However, at 12 months post-vaccination a higher BMI corresponded with a precipitous drop in antibodies.

- Obese adults also had significantly decreased $CD8^+$ T-cell activation and reduced expression of functional proteins versus healthy weight adults.

- Two markers of functional $CD8^+$ activity — granzyme B and interferon gamma — were significantly decreased in the obese adults. ($CD8^+$ T-cells combat virus-infected cells by releasing granzyme B and inhibit viral replication by releasing interferon gamma.)

- Obese adults 1) had a steeper drop in influenza vaccine antibodies over time compared with healthy weight adults, and 2) are deficient in the expression of granzyme B and interferon gamma. These factors indicate that immunity against an influenza infection may be suboptimal in the obese population.

219.

Vaccinated obese adults are at risk of influenza despite high antibody levels

"Despite robust serological responses, vaccinated obese adults are twice as likely to develop influenza and influenza-like illness compared to healthy-weight adults. This finding challenges the current standard for correlates of protection, suggesting use of antibody titers to determine vaccine effectiveness in an obese population may provide misleading information."

Neidich SD, Green WD, et al. **Increased risk of influenza among vaccinated adults who are obese.** *Int J Obes (Lond)* 2017; 41(9): 1324-30.

- Previous studies have shown that obesity increases the risk of influenza-related adverse health outcomes including hospitalization and death.

- This study was conducted to determine whether obese adults vaccinated against influenza have an increased risk of contracting influenza and influenza-like illness (ILI) as compared to vaccinated healthy-weight adults.

- A total of 1022 adults completed the study. Healthy weight was defined as a BMI of 18.5-24.9 and obese as a BMI of ≥ 30.

- Compared with vaccinated healthy-weight adults, vaccinated obese adults had twice the risk of developing influenza or ILI (relative risk, RR = 2.01).

- This study also found that increased susceptibility to influenza and ILI in obese adults was not associated with a failure to achieve "seroprotective" antibody levels: there were no statistical differences in antibody responses between vaccinated healthy-weight and obese adults.

- The increased risk of influenza in the obese population may be due to an impaired T-cell function, despite a robust seroprotective antibody response.

220.

Obese mice have poor immune responses to influenza and covid vaccination

"We herein showed that obese mice vaccinated and then challenged with pandemic 2009 H1N1 virus showed impaired immune responses, uncontrolled inflammation, and increased mortality. These results may have significant public health implications suggesting that conventional vaccine strategies may be less effective in the obese population."

Kim YH, Kim JK, et al. **Diet-induced obesity dramatically reduces the efficacy of a 2009 pandemic H1N1 vaccine in a mouse model.** *J Infect Dis* 2012 Jan 15; 205(2): 244-51.

- This study investigated whether obese mice have altered vaccine-induced immune responses and protective efficacy against the H1N1 influenza virus.

- In obese mice, antibody responses were dramatically reduced. They also had severe lung inflammation, greatly increased expression of proinflammatory cytokines and chemokines in lung tissue, and a 100% mortality rate, compared with a 14% mortality rate in the lean mice.

221.

O'Meara TR, Nanishi E, et al. **Reduced SARS-CoV-2 mRNA vaccine immunogenicity and protection in mice with diet-induced obesity and insulin resistance.** *J Allergy Clin Immunol* 2023 Nov;152(5):1107-1120.e6.

"Our study demonstrates that diet-induced obesity and type-2 diabetes mellitus in a murine model reduce immunogenicity and protective efficacy of the SARS-CoV-2 BNT162b2 [Pfizer] mRNA vaccine."

- Many currently approved vaccines, including mRNA covid vaccines, are not very effective in people with obesity or diabetes.

- In this study, scientists fed mice a high-fat diet until they developed obesity and insulin resistance. Next, they were vaccinated with an mRNA covid vaccine. Compared to mice fed a normal diet, the obese mice developed significantly lower anti-spike IgG titers and a 3.83-fold decrease in neutralizing antibodies.

222.

Obesity significantly increases the risk of severe covid-19 illness requiring hospitalization and intensive care

"Our data indicate that obese subjects may be at higher risk for serious illness if infected and obesity may play a role in the progression of covid-19."

Helvaci N, Eyupoglu ND, et al. **Prevalence of obesity and its impact on outcome in patients with covid-19: a systematic review and meta-analysis.** *Front Endocrinol (Lausanne)* 2021 Feb 25; 12: 598249.

- In this paper, researchers systematically reviewed 19 studies from the United States, Europe and Asia to determine the prevalence of obesity in patients with covid-19, and their risk of severe illness.

- The pooled obesity prevalence rates were 32% in hospitalized patients, 41% in patients admitted to an intensive care unit (ICU), and 43% in patients requiring invasive mechanical ventilation (IMV). All rates were significantly higher than the 13.2% worldwide prevalence of obesity.

- The pooled analysis revealed that covid-19 patients with obesity had a 30% increased risk of being hospitalized (OR = 1.3), a 51% increased risk for ICU admission (OR = 1.51), and a 77% increased risk of requiring IMV (OR = 1.77) compared to non-obese patients.

- In European nations, prevalence rates of obesity in covid-19 patients who died were significantly higher than the background obesity prevalence rates.

- Obesity is a known risk factor for high blood pressure, type 2 diabetes, and cardiovascular disease, comorbidities associated with severe cases of covid-19.

- In patients with covid-19, obesity-induced chronic inflammation and impaired immunity may contribute to severe adverse health outcomes.

- Obesity substantially changes pulmonary mechanics and respiratory muscle function, predisposing patients to respiratory failure during a lung infection.

223.

Nations with the highest proportions of overweight and obese adults have the worst covid-19 death rates

"Covid-19 is only the latest of a series of respiratory viral diseases that have affected human populations. There is every reason to assume that future infectious diseases will follow similar patterns, and that an unhealthy population — i.e. an overweight population — will raise the likelihood of another pandemic."

Lobstein T. **Covid-19 and obesity: the 2021 atlas.** *World Obesity Federation* 2021 Mar: 1-226.

- This report from the World Obesity Foundation analyzed data from 164 nations to determine whether there is an association between covid-19 deaths and body weight. Data was provided by Johns Hopkins University and the World Health Organization.

- Covid-19 death rates were found to be 10 times higher in nations where more than half of the adult population is overweight (BMI $\geq$ 25).

- About 2.2 million of the 2.5 million deaths from covid were in nations with the highest proportions of overweight adults.

- The US, UK, and Italy have exceptionally high percentages of overweight adults in their populations — 68%, 64%, and 59% respectively — and they also have some of the worst covid death rates in the world.

- Nations such as Japan, South Korea, and Vietnam have very low levels of adult obesity and very low covid death rates.

- In the US, where 68% of all adults are overweight, 88% of covid patients requiring intensive care are overweight. Just 12% of covid patients requiring intensive care are normal weight.

- The author of this report warns that "an overweight population is the next pandemic waiting to happen."

224.

Obesity significantly increases the risk of a poor outcome to covid-19

"A healthy lifestyle, particularly achieving ideal body weight, is very important in preventing and reducing a composite poor outcome, including mortality, if a person contracts covid-19."

Soeroto AY, Soetedjo NN, et al. **Effect of increased BMI and obesity on the outcome of Covid-19 adult patients: a systematic review and meta-analysis.** *Diabetes Metab Syndr* 2020 Nov-Dec; 14(6): 1897-1904.

• Obesity leads to a weak immune response to infections, chronic activation of the innate immune system, systemic inflammation, and airway constriction.

• A meta-analysis was conducted utilizing 16 studies to determine if obesity is associated with a poor outcome in adult patients with covid-19.

• Obesity significantly increased the risk of a poor outcome to covid-19 (OR = 1.78, $p < 0.001$). Covid-19 patients with a poor outcome had a higher BMI.

• A subgroup analysis found that obesity was related with other poor outcomes, including hospital admission, severe covid-19, acute respiratory distress syndrome (ARDS), and use of mechanical ventilation (OR = 2.22, $p < 0.001$).

225.

Pellini R, Venuti A, et al. **Initial observations on age, gender, BMI and hypertension in antibody responses to SARS-CoV-2 BNT162b2 vaccine.** *EClinicalMedicine* 2021 Jun; 36: 100928.

"Differences among BMI classes and antibody titres was noticed (p = 0.02)...with higher values in under- and normal-weight groups compared to pre-obesity and obesity groups."

• This study analyzed the antibody titers of 248 healthcare workers (23 to 69 years of age) 7 days after they received the second dose of a covid-19 vaccine.

• Non-parametric analysis yielded $p = 0.033$ for BMI, and $p = 0.0001$ for age.

226.

Obesity is a significant risk factor for severe covid-19

"The findings in this report highlight a dose-response relationship between higher BMI and severe COVID-19-associated illness."

Kompaniyets L, Goodman AB, et al. **Body mass index and risk for COVID-19-related hospitalization, ICU admission, invasive mechanical ventilation, and death—United States, March- December 2020.** *MMWR Morb Mortal Wkly Rep* 2021 Mar 12; 70(10): 355-361.

- In this CDC analysis, the association between body mass index (BMI) and risk for severe covid was assessed. The sample population included 148,494 adults who were diagnosed with covid at 238 U.S. hospitals.

- Obesity significantly increased the risk for hospitalization and death, especially among adults less than 65 years of age. Overweight and obese adults had a significantly higher risk for invasive mechanical ventilation.

227.

Senthilingam M. **Covid-19 has made the obesity epidemic worse, but failed to ignite enough action.** *BMJ* 2021 Mar 4; 372: n411.

"The evidence is clear that obesity is a risk factor for severe covid-19 disease and death."

- This report summarizes studies showing that obesity increases the risk of severe morbidity and death associated with covid-19.

- Studies in the US have shown that obesity increases the risk of covid-related hospital admissions by 113%, intensive care admissions by 74%, and of dying by 48%. In the UK, people with a BMI over 40 have a 90% increased risk of dying from covid-19.

- Obese individuals are also more likely to have poor immune responses to the covid-19 vaccine.

Super-spreaders

Not everyone is equally contagious when they contract an infectious disease. Some people are super-spreaders who infect many people with their illness. Many super-spreaders have a high viral load and shed the virus for a long time. The propensity of individuals to exhale a large quantity of respiratory droplets increases with age and elevated body mass index (obesity). Super-spreaders are also more likely to be asymptomatic males over 40 years of age. Because super-spreaders spread the disease disproportionately, random population-wide approaches to disease control efforts should be reconsidered. Since super-spreading is a normal feature of disease spread, targeting highly infectious individuals is a more effective strategy at controlling outbreaks of disease.

228.

Some people are super-spreaders who infect many people with their illness

"With respect to human borne illnesses, a superspreader is someone who is more likely to infect other humans when compared to a typically infected person."

Mohindra R, Ghai A, et al. **Superspreaders: a lurking danger in the community.** *J Prim Care and Community Health* 2021;12: 2150132720987432.

- Just as all people are not equally susceptible to contracting an infectious disease, some people who are infected with a disease are more contagious than others. These "superspreaders" are likely to infect many people.

- This paper provides examples of people who contracted and spread covid-19 to several other people. It also discusses factors that affect superspreading.

- A 33-year-old male healthcare worker in India who tested positive for covid-19 had direct or indirect contact with 49 people who subsequently became infected, which led to an outbreak of 235 cases in the community.

- A superspreader in New York spread covid-19 to 20 other people in his neighborhood, which ultimately caused a cluster of nearly 100 cases.

- Superspreaders can be asymptomatic or severely ill. They could infect numerous people because they have an increased viral load, prolonged viral shedding, and/or extensive social interactions.

- Disease transmission is influenced by the basic reproductive number, R-naught (the average number of infections caused by typically infectious people) and the individual reproductive number (the actual number of infections caused by specific individuals).

- Diabetes, hypertension, immune disorders, and other co-morbidities may also influence the rate of disease transmission.

- Several studies refer to the 20/80 rule, which suggests that 20% of the people in a population are associated with 80% of the spread of a disease.

229.

Covid super-spreaders tend to be asymptomatic males over 40 years of age

"It has long been noted that for a variety of diseases, 20% of the host population has the potential to cause 80% of transmission."

Brainard J, Jones NR, et al. **Super-spreaders of novel coronaviruses that cause SARS, MERS and COVID-19: a systematic review.** *Ann Epidemiol* 2023 Jun; 82: 66-76.

• Most individuals with coronavirus infections transmit disease to one or two other people, but some individuals are super-spreaders infecting many people.

• The authors reviewed 163 studies. They sought to identify characteristics of these super-spreaders.

• Scientists define super-spreading as "above the average number of secondary cases" or as "the 1% of index cases that generated the most secondary infections."

• The most typical super-spreader was a male at least 40 years of age. Covid super-spreaders were often asymptomatic and spread disease in the community.

230.

Kawahara T, Ueki Y, et al. **Characteristics of SARS-CoV-2 super-spreaders in Japan.** *J Infect* 2022 Feb; 84(2): e6-e9. [Letter.]

• Super-spreaders have a high viral load and shed the virus for a long time.

• In more than 90% of patients who had multiple PCR tests performed, the viral load was its maximum at the first or second test.

• Patients with diabetes, arthritis, and history of stroke were significantly more likely to have a higher copy number, even after adjusting for confounders.

• Findings in this paper can be helpful to identify super-spreaders using knowledge of comorbidities and laboratory information at the time of admission.

231.

Covid super-spreaders may be asymptomatic and are difficult to identify

"The results from these studies suggest that there is some difficulty in detecting COVID-19 super-spreaders, considering that many infected people are asymptomatic."

Rambo APS, Goncalves LF, et al. **Impact of super-spreaders on COVID-19: systematic review.** *Sao Paulo Med J* 2021 Mar-Apr; 139(2): 163-69.

- Super-spreader is a term referring to individuals who have greater potential to infect other people.

- The authors of this paper analyzed four other papers to identify characteristics of covid super-spreaders.

- Although it is difficult to identify and control super-spreaders, it is presumed that they have a high viral load and participate in a social event.

232.

Kumar S, Jha S, Rai SK. **Significance of super spreader events in COVID-19.** *Indian J Public Health* 2020 Jun; 64(Supplement): S139-141.

"An epidemic containment strategy needs to include early identification of super spreaders to limit an explosive growth."

- Most super-spreader events are identified in hindsight. Typhoid Mary was a super-spreader.

- Many super-spreaders have a high viral load and shed more of the virus. They often spread the infection prior to realizing they are infected.

- Super-spreaders often work in or visit crowded places and/or may disregard quarantine instructions.

- It is important to study super-spreaders as a vital aspect of epidemic control.

233.

Elevated age and obesity increase the risk of spreading covid-19

"We observed that 18% of human subjects accounted for 80% of the exhaled bioaerosol of the group, reflecting a super-spreader distribution of bioaerosol analogous to a classical 20:80 super-spreader of infection distribution."

Edwards DA, Ausiello D, et al. **Exhaled aerosol increases with covid-19 infection, age, and obesity.** *PNAS* 2021 Feb 23; 118(8): e2021830118.

- In this paper, scientists studied exhaled respiratory droplets in 194 humans and 8 non-human primates with and without covid-19 infection to assess the quantity and size of exhaled aerosol particles in healthy and diseased subjects.

- The generation of respiratory droplets in exhaled breath occurs when people breathe, talk, cough and sneeze.

- The findings in this paper suggest that the transmissibility of viral matter is related to the propensity of individuals to exhale a large quantity of small respiratory droplets. This propensity increases with the advance of covid-19 infection, age, and elevated body mass index (obesity).

- All of the subjects in the study who were less than 26 years of age and healthy weight were low spreaders of exhaled bioaerosol.

- Elderly and obese individuals (and the obese elderly) are at risk of developing severe symptoms of covid-19 infection and also have a higher probability of expelling the virus into the environment and transmitting the disease.

- The contagiousness of an individual is not only associated with a growth in viral load during infection and the proximity of the infected individual to those who are uninfected, but may be related to phenotype as well.

- Advanced age and obesity may be associated with the phenomenon of super-spreading, which suggests that approximately 20% of infected people are responsible for about 80% of the spread of a disease.

234.

Obese adults shed and potentially spread the influenza virus for a significantly longer duration than non-obese adults

"We found that, even in asymptomatic or mildly ill individuals, obese adults shed influenza A virus for a longer duration than non-obese adults. This has important implications for influenza transmission."

Maier HE, Lopez R, et al. **Obesity increases the duration of influenza A virus shedding in adults.** *J Infect Dis* 2018 Sep 22; 218(9): 1378-82.

- In this paper, researchers investigated the effect of obesity on the duration of viral shedding during influenza infections.

- Since obesity alters immune function and increases mechanical difficulties in breathing, the authors hypothesized that this could lead to a longer duration of influenza virus shedding and increased transmissibility of the infection.

- A total of 1783 people in 320 households were intensively monitored for 10-13 days once an influenza case was identified.

- Symptomatic obese adults shed the influenza A virus 42% longer than non-obese adults (event time ratio, ETR = 1.42; 95% CI, 1.06-1.89).

- Among asymptomatic cases or those with less than 1 symptom (not including fever), obese adults shed the influenza A virus twice as long as non-obese adults (ETR = 2.04; 95% CI, 1.35-3.09).

- No significant relationship was found between obesity and shedding duration for influenza B virus.

- Obesity was defined as a Body Mass Index (BMI) of ≥ 30 in adults.

235.

Super-spreaders have high viral loads which could generate new super-spreaders

"Infections caused by contact with super-spreaders are more likely to result in new super-spreaders than those caused by transmission from a less infectious individual."

Beldomenico PM. **Do superspreaders generate new superspreaders? A hypothesis to explain the propagation pattern of COVID-19.** *Int J Infect Dis* 2020 Jul; 96: 461-63.

- During the early stages of the covid pandemic, data revealed that a small number of covid cases were responsible for most transmissions of the disease.

- Super-spreaders may have high viral shedding and active social behavior.

- Super-spreaders might generate new super-spreaders by exposing people to elevated viral loads. This type of infectious transmission should be considered during disease mitigation campaigns.

236.

Al-Tawfiq JA, Rodriguez-Morales AJ. **Super-spreading events and contribution to transmission of MERS, SARS, and SARS-CoV-2 (COVID-19).** *J Hosp Infect* 2020 Jun; 105(2): 111-112.

"There are multiple explanations for the occurrence of super-spreading events, including immune suppression, increased disease severity and viral load, asymptomatic individuals, and extensive social interactions."

- Individuals with severe disease may have higher viral loads and are more likely to spread higher infectious doses.

- Individuals with a higher viral load and more environmental contacts could disproportionately contribute to super-spreading events.

237.

Disease control efforts should be directed at highly infectious super-spreaders rather than at random people

"Heterogeneous infectiousness, and its extreme manifestation of super-spreading, are likely to be general properties of disease transmission in populations. The ambitious aim of controlling disease emergence will require a better understanding of those properties."

Galvani AP, May RM. **Epidemiology: dimensions of superspreading.** *Nature* 2005 Nov 17; 438(7066): 293-95.

- Individuals were originally treated as having an equal chance of transmitting disease. Variations in transmission capability, or heterogeneous infectiousness and the disproportionate influence of super-spreaders, was largely ignored.

- Disease control efforts should identify the highly infectious super-spreaders and target interventions at them. Thus, outbreaks may be halted sooner, with fewer people treated, than if efforts are directed at random people.

238.

Bouayed J, Bohn T. **Behavioral manipulation—key to the successful global spread of the new coronavirus SARS CoV 2?** *J Med Virol* 2021 Mar; 93(3): 1748-51.

"This should address the question whether there exists a close relationship between higher viral load and the manipulative ability of the virus."

- During the covid pandemic, irresponsible behavior in covid-infected individuals, mostly in super-spreaders, was reported. Some infected people ignored self-confinement and physical distancing while increasing social interactions.

- This paper highlights the possibility that covid infections alter human social behavior to benefit covid transmission. Research should focus on the psychology of individuals to determine whether their personality traits are predisposed to manipulation by the covid virus.

239.

Targeting highly infectious individuals is more effective at disease control than population-wide approaches

"Our findings show that emerging disease outbreaks cannot be fully understood if individual variation in infectiousness is neglected."

Lloyd-Smith JO, Schreiber SJ, et al. **Superspreading and the effect of individual variation on disease emergence.** *Nature* 2005 Nov 17; 438(7066): 355-59.

- R-naught (R0) refers to the mean number of infections caused by an infected person. However, population estimates of R0 don't account for individual variation in infectiousness, or super-spreading events, in which certain people infect many other people.

- Predictions that factor in individual infectiveness differ from population-wide approaches. Outbreaks are more rare and disease extinction is more likely.

- Super-spreading is a normal feature of disease spread. Focusing half of all control effort on the most infectious cases is up to three times more effective than random population-wide control.

240.

Kemper JT. **On the identification of superspreaders for infectious disease.** *Mathematical Biosciences* 1980; 48: 111-127.

"Through increased understanding of the role played by super-spreaders, more informed decisions can be made concerning the type of data which must be considered in any discussion of their existence or effect."

- Although in 1980 researchers were not yet able to precisely identify super-spreaders, the author provides mathematical models hypothesizing their effect on disease occurrence.

241.

Super-spreaders were originally referred to as dangerous carriers

"The term super-spreader was first coined in 1972, in relation to stochastic computer simulations of influenza epidemics."

Teicher A. **Super-spreaders: a historical review.** *Lancet Infect Dis* 2023 Oct; 23(10): e409-e417.

- The author reviews the history of the super-spreader concept.

- During the early 20th century, super-spreaders were originally called "dangerous carriers" associated with gastrointestinal ailments, not respiratory ones.

- Other early terms for super-spreader were dangerous transmitters, dangerous disseminators, and dangerous habitual spreaders.

- During the 1957-58 influenza pandemic, a greater awareness of airborne transmission and wide variability in infectiousness became more established.

- In the 1970s and 1980s, the term was used to explain why outbreaks of airborne diseases occurred in vaccinated populations.

- During the 1980s, the term was associated with sexually transmitted infections.

- Today, a carrier might be seen as dangerous due to behavioral or immunological factors, especially asymptomatic carriers unaware of their infection.

- Some researchers prefer to speak about super-spreading events rather than people, to shift the stigma from individuals to environmental factors.

Measles and MMR

The measles and MMR vaccines have been associated with several adverse effects. For example, Hooker found that children who received their first MMR vaccine before 36 months of age were significantly more likely to receive an autism diagnosis when compared to children who received their first MMR at a later age. This effect was much more pronounced in Black males. Measles and MMR have also been associated with encephalopathy, brain damage, and death. The National Childhood Vaccine Injury Act presumes vaccine causation if encephalopathy occurs within 15 days after measles or MMR vaccination. The Institute of Medicine also has acknowledged biologic plausibility.

In China, most children receive two doses of the measles vaccine and in some urban areas they receive three doses. Yet, a substantial number of vaccinated children contract the disease. During a measles outbreak in California, many of the suspected cases occurred in people who were recently vaccinated against measles. Of the 194 measles viruses genetically analyzed in the U.S. that year, 73 (37.6%) were identified as vaccine strains. Thus, fully vaccinated children are still susceptible to the disease.

Several studies by Aaby and colleagues contradict previous studies that suggested wild measles is associated with delayed excess mortality. Studies conducted in Senegal, Guinea-Bissau, and Bangladesh showed that children who contracted measles had lower mortality when compared to unvaccinated children who did not contract measles. Post-measles cases had lower all-cause mortality than controls. Thus, the assumption that measles is associated with delayed excess mortality after the acute phase of infection due to long-term immune suppression, and that this post-measles mortality could be averted by vaccination, may not be true.

242.

Black male children have a higher risk of autism when receiving MMR before 3 years of age

"Black males...appear to be 38% more likely to receive an autism diagnosis if they received the first MMR vaccine one year earlier than the controls. The effect originally observed by the CDC and affirmed in this paper, showing a greater risk specifically for African-Americans, deserves additional, immediate investigation."

Hooker BS. **Reanalysis of CDC data on autism incidence and time of first MMR vaccination.** *Journal of American Physicians and Surgeons* 2018 Winter; 23(4): 105-9.

- In 2004, the CDC published a paper in which children with autism were significantly more likely to have received an MMR vaccine before 36 months of age when compared to a control group of children who did not have autism (odds ratio, OR = 1.49). Boys had an even higher risk (OR = 1.67).

- In this current paper, CDC data from the earlier study was re-analyzed with a focus on race and gender, examining autism rates in African-American and white children based on the age when MMR was initially administered.

- Black males who received their first MMR vaccine before 36 months of age were nearly 4 times more likely to be diagnosed with autism when compared to black males who received their first MMR at a later age (OR = 3.86).

- All children (regardless of race or gender) who received their first MMR vaccine before 36 months of age were significantly more likely to receive "an autism diagnosis without mental retardation" when compared to all children who received their first MMR at a later age (OR = 2.52).

- Infant vaccines contained much more mercury starting in 1990. Black males born in 1990 or later had higher rates of autism than black males born earlier. These results suggest the possibility of a synergism between early mercury exposure (not from MMR) and MMR timing leading to a greater risk of autism.

- The CDC appeared to conceal MMR-autism findings on black males.

243.

Measles and MMR vaccines may cause encephalopathy followed by permanent brain damage and death

"In the absence of any obvious bias and confounding, this finding is evidence for a causal relationship between further attenuated measles vaccine, alone or in combination, and acute encephalopathy of undetermined cause followed by permanent brain impairment or death."

Weibel RE, Caserta V, et al. **Acute encephalopathy followed by permanent brain injury or death associated with further attenuated measles vaccines: a review of claims submitted to the National Vaccine Injury Compensation Program.** *Pediatrics* 1998 Mar; 101(3 Pt 1): 383-7.

- In this paper, claims submitted to the National Vaccine Injury Compensation Program were reviewed to determine if there is evidence for a causal relationship between receipt of a measles, mumps, rubella, or MMR vaccine and acute encephalopathy followed by permanent brain injury or death.

- Medical records of children who met the inclusion criteria and developed encephalopathy within 15 days following vaccination were analyzed.

- Forty-eight children met the inclusion criteria and developed encephalopathy of undetermined cause after receiving a measles or MMR vaccine. Eight (16.7%) of the children died; the remainder had mental regression, retardation, chronic seizures, behavioral changes, sensory deficits, and motor disorders.

- A statistically significant non-random clustering of encephalopathy cases occurred on days 8 and 9 after measles or MMR vaccination, indicative of causation. Mumps and rubella vaccines were not associated with encephalitis.

- The National Childhood Vaccine Injury Act presumes vaccine causation if encephalopathy occurs within 15 days after measles or MMR vaccination. The Institute of Medicine also has acknowledged biologic plausibility.

- The patients had a median age of 15 months and a mean age of 17.5 months. The 48 cases were likely under-reported because the passive system does not require filing for compensation and medical documentation is required.

244.

Neurologic disorders, including encephalopathy and convulsions, are possible following measles vaccination

"Causes of these cases [of encephalopathy] could not be established, but 45 (76%) had onset between 6 and 15 days after measles vaccination; this clustering suggests that some may have been caused by vaccine."

Landrigan PJ, Witte JJ. **Neurologic disorders following live measles-virus vaccination.** *JAMA* 1973 Mar 26; 223(13): 1459-62.

- Fifty-nine of 84 patients developed encephalopathy after measles vaccination. Eleven of the cases were febrile convulsions. At least 5 of the patients died.

245.

Millson DS. **Brother-to-sister transmission of measles after measles, mumps, and rubella immunisation.** *Lancet* 1989; 1(8632): 271. [Letter.]

- A healthy 4-year-old boy received an MMR vaccine and developed symptoms of measles after 10 days. A few days later, his unvaccinated 8-month-old sister developed almost clinically identical symptoms of measles.

- This case study provides evidence that children who were recently vaccinated with MMR may transmit measles to other children.

246.

Washam MC, Leber AL, et al. **Shedding of measles vaccine RNA in children after receiving measles, mumps and rubella vaccination.** *J Clin Virol* 2024 August; 174: 105696.

"Shedding of measles vaccine RNA is not uncommon and vaccine RNA can be detected up to 29 days post MMR."

- Ninety-six nasopharyngeal samples were collected from children after the first dose of MMR, of which 33 (34.4%) were positive for vaccine RNA.

247.

Fully vaccinated children
are still susceptible to measles

*"Public health officials in China are concerned about the high number
of measles cases among individuals with multiple vaccinations."*

Masters NB, Wagner AL, et al. **Assessing measles vaccine failure in Tianjin,
China.** *Vaccine* 2019 May 31; 37(25): 3251-54.

- In China, most children receive two doses of the measles vaccine. Yet, a substantial number of vaccinated children contract the disease.

- The median time from vaccination (at least two doses) to a diagnosis of measles was 4.26 years. The shortest time was 1.33 years.

- The onset of measles for children who received only one dose of the measles vaccine was similar to unvaccinated children.

248.

Yang W, Li J, Shaman J. **Characteristics of measles epidemics in China
(1951-2004) and implications for elimination: A case study of three key
locations.** *PLoS Comput Biol* 2019 Feb 4; 15(2): e1006806.

*"In China, where countrywide vaccination coverage for the last
decade has been above 95% (the threshold for measles elimination),
measles continues to cause large epidemics."*

- In China, which holds 18% of the world's population, vaccination rates have been above 95% for the past decade yet measles epidemics continue to occur.

- The dynamics of measles transmission are complex, influenced by population susceptibility related to birth rates, death rates, migration, natural infection, vaccination, and contact patterns, such as mixing of populations in schools.

- This study estimated that to eliminate measles in China with a vaccine that provides 95% efficacy, 98.7% of the population must be vaccinated.

249.

Vaccine-induced immunity in populations without wild measles is insufficient to prevent susceptibility to the disease

"Waning levels of measles antibodies with increasing time post-vaccination suggests that measles susceptibility is potentially increasing in Korea. This trend may be related to limitations of vaccine-induced immunity in the absence of natural boosting by the wild virus, compared to naturally acquired immunity triggered by measles infection."

Kang HJ, Han YW, et al. **An increasing, potentially measles-susceptible population over time after vaccination in Korea.** *Vaccine* 2017 Jul 24; 35(33): 4126-32.

- In South Korea, the 2-dose MMR vaccination coverage rate has been maintained at greater than 95% since 1996. Yet measles cases have occurred in infants and fully vaccinated 13-24-year-olds.

- In this paper, scientists analyzed measles antibody levels in 3050 healthy Koreans to assess the degree of measles susceptibility in Korea.

- Children 1-6 years of age had the highest prevalence of antibodies against measles at 93%. Adolescents 16-19 years of age had the lowest at 48.5%. Measles seropositivity gradually decreased from 100% in children 5-6 years of age to 42% in 19-year-olds.

- Infants 1 month of age had passive immunity (from maternal antibodies) of 76%, which decreased to 8% by 3 months of age. As more women acquire immunity by vaccination instead of natural measles infection, early waning of vaccine-induced maternal antibodies places more infants at risk of measles.

- This study found that 1) measles antibody titers decreased with increasing time post-vaccination, and 2) the proportion of the population with a low antibody titer was greater in the current year when compared to a previous study conducted four years earlier.

- From 2010-2016, among all individuals with confirmed measles infections, 47% were vaccinated (36% with 2 doses) and 36% were unvaccinated.

250.

Vaccine strains of measles can be genetically distinguished from wild strains despite causing similar symptoms

"During measles outbreaks, it is important to be able to rapidly distinguish between measles cases and vaccine reactions."

Roy F, Mendoza L, et al. **Rapid identification of measles virus vaccine genotype by real-time PCR.** *J Clin Microbiol* 2017 Mar; 55(3): 735-43.

- Although measles was nearly eliminated in the Americas in 2002, large outbreaks still occur.

- About 5% of people vaccinated against measles develop symptoms similar to wild measles. It is essential to quickly identify vaccine reactions from actual cases of the disease so that labor-intensive health measures, such as contact tracing, can be avoided and patients with vaccine reactions are not isolated.

- This paper discusses the development of a real-time reverse transcription method (MeVA RT-qPCR) that can rapidly differentiate between adverse reactions caused by measles vaccine strains and wild strains of the disease.

- The World Health Organization (WHO) recognizes 24 genotypes of the measles virus. All of the vaccine strains belong to genotype A. Wild measles viruses of genotype A are no longer circulating.

- During a measles outbreak in California in 2015, many of the suspected cases occurred in people who were recently vaccinated against measles. Of the 194 measles viruses genetically analyzed in the U.S. that year, 73 (37.6%) were identified as vaccine strains.

- Genotyping is used to determine the origin of a measles outbreak and is the only way to distinguish vaccine strains from wild viruses. However, when the RT-qPCR was tested at three global laboratories, one wild genotype (D5) gave a false positive and 3 of 88 genotype A samples went undetected.

- Measles cases are determined by genotype, not symptoms. If the symptoms are caused by a vaccine strain, then it's not a case but a vaccine reaction.

251.

A new measles sub-strain that is resistant to neutralizing antibodies has emerged in nations with high vaccination rates

"Because measles vaccination with a genetically restricted strain (genotype A) has been used throughout the world for 50 years, changes in genotype circulation patterns might reflect the immune selection of 'fitter' viruses."

Muñoz-Alía MÁ, Muller CP, Russell SJ. **Antigenic drift defines a new D4 subgenotype of measles virus.** *J Virol* 2017 May 12; 91(11): e00209-17.

- Health authorities planned to eliminate measles by 2020 through increased vaccination rates. However, officials are concerned that measles cases among vaccinated people due to waning immunity and antigenic shifts in circulating strains might prevent the eradication of measles from ever being achieved.

- The wild measles virus possesses hemagglutinin protein that binds with cells and causes infection. The measles vaccine protects against infection by inducing antibodies that neutralize the function of the hemagglutinin protein.

- There are 24 genotypes associated with the measles virus. In this study, the authors examined the D4 strain and describe two newly emerged variants: sub-genotypes D4.1 and D4.2.

- The D4.2 sub-genotype, which was found predominantly in France and Great Britain — countries with high vaccination rates — showed resistance to neutralizing antibodies, suggesting that extensive vaccination might provide an environment conducive to selective pressure and adaptive mutations.

- Newly emerged sub-genotype D4.2 measles viruses were not counteracted by antibodies targeting them, and infection was unhampered.

- The World Health Organization affirms that the D4 genotype currently represents about 20% of measles viruses reported in databases, a high prevalence.

- Evidence presented in this paper indicates that a single point mutation is sufficient for the measles virus to escape neutralizing antibodies.

252.

Circulating strains of measles have mutated causing outbreaks of measles despite a high measles vaccination rate

"These data suggest that the increased incidence of measles in Jilin Province may be attributed to the antigenic drift between wild-type and vaccine strains."

Shi J, Zheng J, et al. **Measles incidence rate and a phylogenetic study of contemporary genotype H1 measles strains in China: is an improved measles vaccine needed?** *Virus Genes* 2011 Dec; 43(3): 319-26.

- In China, primary vaccine failure and measles outbreaks still occur although more than 98.5% of all infants are vaccinated, indicating that measles vaccines may not be effective against circulating strains. Without investigating, it is unknown whether wild measles viruses have drifted away from the vaccine.

- This study investigated the genetic variation of wild-type measles strains and compared their nucleoprotein (N) and hemagglutinin (H) genes with two existing genotype A vaccine strains.

- The variation rate between the vaccine and wild-type strains was 9.8-12% in the N gene and 5.9-6.9% in the H gene, respectively. In addition, the sera obtained from infants following primary vaccination decreased 4-fold in its capacity to neutralize wild-type measles virus isolates.

- Findings in this paper suggest that mutations of the wild-type measles virus, and antigenic drift between wild-type and vaccine strains, may be a factor causing increased outbreaks of measles despite high vaccination rates.

- Although measles is believed to be a single serotype, genetic variability occurs in wild strains, and existing vaccines may be unable to protect populations from measles mutations.

- New measles vaccines may be required to neutralize circulating strains of wild-type measles viruses more effectively, to overcome primary vaccine failure and avert measles outbreaks.

253.

Natural measles confers long-term protection against fatal infections

"Contrary to current assumptions, children who survive the acute phase of measles infection may have a survival advantage compared with unimmunized, uninfected children.... The possibility that infections could have beneficial effects raises questions about the value of eradication strategies."

Aaby P. **Assumptions and contradictions in measles and measles immunization research: is measles good for something?** *Soc Sci Med* 1995 Sep; 41(5): 673-86.

- This paper reviewed studies that determined causal factors associated with acute measles case fatality rates, the delayed impact of measles, and mortality after measles vaccination.

- The mortality rate is much higher in people who contract measles at home compared to those who are infected from someone outside the home. This may be related to the intensity or amplification of exposure. Index (or first) cases were found to have 3 times lower mortality than secondary cases.

- Measles is more severe when contracted from the opposite sex, and mortality is higher in homes where a boy and girl are simultaneously infected.

- Studies conducted in Senegal, Guinea-Bissau, and Bangladesh showed that children who contracted measles had lower mortality when compared to unvaccinated children who did not contract measles. Studies from Tanzania found that measles reduced the prevalence and severity of malaria.

- A Danish study found that adults with no history of measles in childhood were 4 times more likely to develop cancers and immune diseases.

- Natural measles and measles vaccination provide a non-specific beneficial effect that increases long-term resistance to other infections.

- Infections can be beneficial. There is no simple answer to how many deaths are associated with measles and how many lives can be saved by vaccination.

254.

Children who contract measles do not have long-term excess mortality due to suppressed immunity

"The authors conclude that measles infection was not associated with increased mortality after the acute phase of infection and that index cases had lower mortality than uninfected, unvaccinated children."

Aaby P, Samb B, et al. **No long-term excess mortality after measles infection: a community study from Senegal.** *Am J Epidemiol* 1996 May 15; 143(10): 1035-41.

- Previous studies in developing countries have shown that measles vaccination reduces overall childhood mortality beyond deaths from acute measles. This extra benefit from vaccination was attributed to the prevention of long-term suppressed immunity presumed to occur after a wild measles infection.

- There was no excess mortality in the post-measles groups compared with unvaccinated children without a history of measles. (mortality ratio, MR = 0.27, 95% CI 0.09-0.85). Findings in this study contradict previous studies that suggested wild measles is associated with delayed excess mortality.

255.

Aaby P, Lisse IM, et al. **No persistent T lymphocyte immunosuppression or increased mortality after measles infection: a community study from Guinea-Bissau.** *Pediatr Infect Dis J* 1996 Jan; 15(1): 39-44.

"There is no indication of persistent suppression of T cell subsets after measles infection, and post-measles cases did not have higher mortality than uninfected community controls."

- Vaccination against measles has reduced overall child mortality, so some researchers have surmised that children who contract wild measles might have excess mortality, due to immunosuppression after a measles infection.

- Post-measles cases had lower all-cause mortality than controls (adjusted mortality rate ratio, MRR = 0.50, 95% CI 0.22-1.16).

256.

Children with measles gain protective benefits against long-term mortality

"When measles infection is mild, clinical measles has no long-term excess mortality and may be associated with better overall survival than no clinical measles infection."

Aaby P, Simondon F, et al. **Low mortality after mild measles infection compared to uninfected children in rural West Africa.** *Vaccine* 2002 Nov 22; 21(1-2): 120-6.

- The assumption that measles is associated with delayed excess mortality after the acute phase of infection due to long-term immune suppression, and that this post-measles mortality could be averted by vaccination, may not be true.

- This study of rural west African children was conducted to assess long-term mortality following a measles epidemic to determine whether mild measles has a beneficial effect, as hypothesized by the study scientists.

- This study found that children with clinical or subclinical measles had significantly lower mortality than children who did not contract measles (mortality ratio, MR = 0.20, 95% CI 0.06-0.74).

- During the 4-year follow-up, 1 of 66 measles cases died (1.5%) whereas 15 of 149 children without measles died (10.1%).

- All of the uninfected children who died were boys while all of the clinical and subclinical measles cases were girls. All deaths during the follow-up were caused by infections, not acute measles.

- The authors also classified children according to intensity of exposure to measles. Children intensively exposed to measles, or exposed early in life, may be more likely to die during the post-measles period. Secondary cases are also more likely to suffer long-term excess mortality than index cases.

- The study authors correctly predicted that the overall effect of measles could be beneficial during outbreaks with low acute measles mortality, when there would be no selection of strong survivors.

DTP and All-Cause Mortality

In many nations, the more reactogenic whole-cell DTP (diphtheria-tetanus-pertussis) vaccine is given to infants and children rather than the acellular DTaP vaccine. Several studies show that DTP-vaccinated children were significantly more likely to die when compared to DTP-unvaccinated children, and girls are more susceptible than boys. In the main analysis of one study of 1057 children, 3-5-month-old infants were 10 times less likely to survive when they were vaccinated against DTP compared to DTP-unvaccinated infants.

Vaccines are designed to prevent specific diseases. However, they also have non-specific effects (NSEs) that either increase or decrease susceptibility to fatal infections not targeted by the vaccine. DTP has negative NSEs that increase all-cause mortality while measles has positive NSEs that decrease all-cause deaths. The last vaccine administered exerts the strongest effect.

In one study that looked at the sequence in which vaccines are administered, children were more than twice as likely to die when they had received DTP with or after a measles vaccine compared with children who had received DTP before a measles vaccine. Girls who received a combination vaccine containing DTP, Hib, and hepatitis B out of sequence were five times more likely to die from all causes within six months of follow-up when compared with girls who received vaccines in the recommended sequence. All currently available evidence suggests that the DTP vaccine may kill more children from other causes than it saves from diphtheria, tetanus or pertussis.

197

257.

DTP-vaccinated children are significantly less likely to survive when compared with DTP-unvaccinated children

"Although lower mortality was expected for DTP-vaccinated children compared with the frail unvaccinated children, DTP vaccination was associated with higher mortality, particularly in girls."

Aaby P, Mogensen SW, et al. **Evidence of increase in mortality after the introduction of diphtheria-tetanus-pertussis vaccine to children aged 6-35 months in Guinea-Bissau: a time for reflection?** *Front Public Health* 2018 Mar 19; 6: 79.

- In 1981, a diphtheria-tetanus-pertussis (DTP) vaccination program was initiated in Guinea-Bissau. Previous studies analyzed the impact of DTP vaccination on all-cause mortality in 3-5-month-old infants. This current study analyzed the effect of DTP on mortality in 6-35-month-old children.

- In the three main analyses in which DTP-vaccinated children had better nutritional status and were protected against three infections — diphtheria, tetanus, and pertussis — they tended to have higher all-cause mortality than the sickly and malnourished DTP-unvaccinated children.

- In a sensitivity analysis, DTP-vaccinated children were significantly less likely to survive compared to DTP-unvaccinated children (hazard ratio, HR = 1.89). DTP-vaccinated girls were nearly 3 times more likely to die (HR = 2.76). Girls did not have higher mortality than boys pre-vaccination.

- The authors also conducted a meta-analysis that included all studies that tested the effect of DTP on mortality in Guinea-Bissau. DTP-vaccinated children were significantly more likely to die when compared to DTP-unvaccinated children (HR = 2.14). The hazard ratio for girls was 2.60.

- Vaccination is usually delayed in unhealthy children, so DTP-unvaccinated children should have had a higher mortality than vaccinated children.

- The World Health Organization is aware of the data indicating that DTP has negative effects increasing mortality but believes the risk is exaggerated.

258.

Infant mortality is 10 times higher in DTP-vaccinated infants compared with DTP-unvaccinated infants

"All currently available evidence suggests that DTP vaccine may kill more children from other causes than it saves from diphtheria, tetanus or pertussis."

Mogensen SW, Andersen A, et al. **The introduction of diphtheria-tetanus-pertussis and oral polio vaccine among young infants in an urban African community: a natural experiment.** *EbioMedicine* 2017 Mar; 17: 192-98.

- Vaccines are designed to protect against specific diseases but may have non-specific effects that increase susceptibility to unrelated infections. Few studies have tested vaccinations for their impact on all-cause mortality.

- In the early 1980s, health authorities introduced diphtheria-tetanus-pertussis (DTP) and oral polio (OPV) vaccines in an urban community in Guinea-Bissau. Scientists analyzed data from that vaccination campaign to compare all-cause mortality among DTP-vaccinated and DTP-unvaccinated infants.

- In the main analysis of 1057 children, 3-5-month-old infants were 10 times less likely to survive when they were vaccinated against DTP compared to DTP-unvaccinated infants (hazard ratio, HR = 10.0).

- Infants were 5 times less likely to survive if they had received DTP plus OPV. (The beneficial non-specific effects of OPV may have reduced the negative non-specific effects of DTP.)

- The DTP-vaccinated and DTP-unvaccinated infants were all from the same cohort of children born in Bandim, Guinea-Bissau. There were no discernible differences in background factors and sick children were not vaccinated.

- In the secondary analysis of 2495 children, the infant mortality rate among infants 3-12 months of age doubled from 1980, before vaccinations, to 1982-1983, after DTP and OPV were introduced (HR = 2.12).

- Most previous studies probably underestimated the detrimental effect of DTP.

259.

In nations with high mortality, the DTP vaccine has non-specific effects that significantly increase the death rate

"DTP is associated with an increase in overall mortality, the effect being particularly negative for girls."

Aaby P, Benn C, et al. **Testing the hypothesis that diphtheria-tetanus-pertussis vaccine has negative non-specific and sex-differential effects on child survival in high-mortality countries.** *BMJ Open* 2012 May 22; 2(3): e000707.

- Vaccines have non-specific effects (NSEs) that can increase or decrease mortality from infectious diseases not targeted by the vaccine. Previous studies have shown that the BCG vaccine (for tuberculosis) and measles vaccine have NSEs that lower all-cause mortality while DTP increases mortality.

- In this paper, scientists tested six hypotheses to verify whether DTP increases mortality. To test these hypotheses, 35 unbiased studies were analyzed.

- All studies without survival bias confirmed that DTP-vaccinated children had significantly higher mortality than DTP-unvaccinated children.

- The order in which vaccines are administered is important. The most recent vaccine given seems to exert the strongest beneficial or detrimental NSE. For example, one study found that mortality was low after BCG, increased after DTP, and dropped again after measles vaccination.

- When children receive DTP *after* a measles vaccine, all-cause mortality increases, and this effect is significantly stronger in girls than boys.

- In this paper, scientists also conducted two randomized studies that reduced the amount of time that DTP would be the last vaccine administered to babies. Both studies suggested that mortality rates would improve by giving a live vaccine — BCG or measles — as soon as possible after DTP.

- Global health officials do not test the sequence of recommended vaccines nor their NSEs to confirm they provide the intended effects on child survival.

260.

Childhood deaths substantially rise when DTP is administered with or after measles vaccination

"The present study found two-fold higher mortality for children receiving DTP with or after measles vaccine."

Aaby P, Biai S, et al. **DTP with or after measles vaccination is associated with increased in-hospital mortality in Guinea-Bissau.** *Vaccine* 2007 Jan 26; 25(7): 1265-69.

- In Guinea-Bissau, DTP is normally given to babies at 6, 10, and 14 weeks of age and the measles vaccine at 9 months. However, it is not uncommon for babies to receive their third dose of DTP out of sequence — concurrently with, or after, measles vaccine.

- In this study, researchers investigated whether DTP administered with or after measles vaccination affected all-cause hospital mortality in children 6-17 months of age.

- Children were more than twice as likely to die when they had received DTP with or after a measles vaccine compared with children who had received a measles vaccine as the last vaccine (case fatality ratio, CFR = 2.53).

- It was common for some children to receive 2 doses of measles vaccine. These children were 5 times more likely to die if they had received DTP after one of the 2 doses of measles vaccine (CFR = 5.62).

- There was no difference in nutritional status among children who received DTP with or after measles vaccine compared with other children.

- The sequence in which vaccines are administered was never evaluated prior to their introduction to determine their impact on all-cause mortality.

- International health organizations quantify the success of national vaccine programs by how many children receive a third dose of DTP. Missing doses are administered out of sequence through catch-up campaigns, causing more children to receive DTP with or after measles vaccine.

261.

Child mortality significantly increases when DTP is given simultaneously with or after measles vaccination

"At 5-8 months of age, essentially all dead children had received DTP as the last vaccination."

Aaby P, Jensen H, Walraven G. **Age-specific changes in the female-male mortality ratio related to the pattern of vaccinations: an observational study from rural Gambia.** *Vaccine* 2006 May 29; 24(22): 4701-8.

- In this study, scientists analyzed data on 537 children less than 5 years of age who died in rural Gambia to determine whether inactivated vaccines, such as DTP, increase female mortality.

- Children who received their third DTP *after* a measles vaccine were significantly more likely to die than children who did not receive DTP as their last vaccine (relative risk, RR = 2.61). Girls had an even higher risk (RR = 3.34).

- Children who received their third DTP *simultaneously* with a measles vaccine were 5 times more likely to die than children who received a measles vaccine only (RR = 5.59). Boys had an even greater risk (RR = 11.61).

262.

Aaby P, Ibrahim SA, et al. **The sequence of vaccinations and increased female mortality after high-titre measles vaccine: trials from rural Sudan and Kinshasa.** *Vaccine* 2006 Apr 5; 24(15): 2764-71.

- In Kinshasa, Congo, children who received their third DTP simultaneously with a measles vaccine died at a rate 5 times higher than children who received a measles vaccine only (mortality rate ratio, MRR = 5.38).

- Studies from Sudan and Congo provide evidence that excess female mortality was due to DTP given at the same time as, or after, measles vaccination.

- Health authorities must consider potential non-specific effects on mortality associated with the sequence in which vaccinations are administered.

263.

DTP-vaccinated girls have 2½ times higher mortality compared with DTP-unvaccinated girls

"Girls are likely to have higher mortality if they are DTP-vaccinated rather than DTP-unvaccinated, and DTP-vaccinated girls are likely to have higher mortality than DTP-vaccinated boys."

Aaby P, Ravn H, et al. **Is diphtheria-tetanus-pertussis (DTP) associated with increased female mortality? A meta-analysis testing the hypotheses of sex-differential non-specific effects of DTP vaccine.** *Trans R Soc Trop Med Hyg* 2016 Dec: 110(10): 570-81.

- Millions of infants throughout the world are required to receive three doses of a whole-cell diphtheria-tetanus-pertussis (DTP) vaccine. Several studies have shown that DTP vaccination increases mortality in girls but the World Health Organization (WHO) claimed the evidence was inconsistent.

- In this paper, all pertinent evidence associated with DTP vaccination and mortality in girls was analyzed, including studies reviewed by WHO, to determine whether differences in methodology, including the choice of studies reviewed, could explain WHO's stance.

- Studies reviewed by WHO used incorrect methodologies which introduced frailty bias and survival bias into the analysis. Deaths were misclassified yielding false findings. These studies should have been excluded from review.

- In this paper, a meta-analysis was conducted with seven studies that used proper methodologies. DTP-vaccinated girls had significantly higher mortality than DTP-unvaccinated girls (mortality rate ratio, MRR = 2.54).

- In a meta-analysis utilizing 10 studies, DTP-vaccinated girls had significantly higher mortality than DTP-vaccinated boys (female/male MRR = 2.45).

- This paper confirms that DTP vaccination in girls induces non-specific effects that are linked with significantly higher mortality from causes other than diphtheria, tetanus, or pertussis as compared with DTP-unvaccinated girls.

264.

Girls are 5 times more likely to die when they receive DTP out of sequence

"It is assumed that providing missing vaccine doses will always leave the child better off than not providing them. This may be wrong."

Fisker AB, Thysen SM. **Non-live pentavalent vaccines after live measles vaccine may increase mortality.** _Vaccine_ 2018 Oct 1; 36(41): 6039-42.

- Vaccines are designed to prevent specific diseases. However, they also have non-specific effects (NSEs) that either increase or decrease susceptibility to potentially fatal infections not targeted by the vaccine.

- The most recent vaccine received exerts the strongest NSEs. Thus, vaccines with known detrimental NSEs (e.g., non-live vaccines such as DTP) should not be given with, or after, vaccines that provide beneficial NSEs.

- In Guinea-Bissau, the pentavalent vaccine (DTP-Hib-hepatitis B) is usually administered at 6, 10, and 14 weeks of age, and the measles vaccine at 9 months. However, delays frequently cause the third pentavalent vaccine to be given concurrently with, or after, measles vaccination.

- This study compared all-cause mortality in children who received vaccines in the recommended sequence (three pentavalent vaccines _before_ measles vaccination) to children who received vaccines out of sequence (the third pentavalent vaccine concurrently with, or after, measles vaccination).

- Children who received a pentavalent vaccine out of sequence were nearly twice as likely to die from all causes by age 5 when compared with children who received vaccines in sequence.

- Girls who received a pentavalent vaccine out of sequence were 5 times more likely to die from all causes within 6 months of follow-up when compared with girls who received vaccines in sequence (hazard ratio, HR = 5.10).

- The sequence of vaccines affects all-cause mortality. The findings in this paper are consistent with previous studies showing higher mortality when DTP is administered simultaneously with, or after, measles vaccination.

265.

DTP and inactivated polio vaccines (IPV) significantly increase female mortality when given after measles vaccination

"Both the observational studies and the randomized trials suggest an increase in overall female mortality in low-income countries for inactivated vaccines administered after measles vaccine."

Aaby P, Ravn H, et al. **Randomized trials comparing inactivated vaccine after medium- or high-titer measles vaccine with standard titer measles vaccine after inactivated vaccine: a meta-analysis.** *Pediatr Infect Dis J* 2016 Nov; 35(11): 1232-41.

- Earlier studies compared a standard measles vaccine given at 9 months of age with a high-titer measles vaccine (HT) given at 5 months of age and concluded that HT was linked with high mortality in girls. Recent studies suggest the high mortality was related to inactivated vaccines given after HT.

- In this paper, scientists conducted a meta-analysis by reanalyzing several earlier studies in Senegal, Guinea-Bissau, Gambia and Sudan to determine whether inactivated vaccines, mainly DTP and IPV, were associated with high mortality, and whether the pattern differed for girls and boys.

- Girls who received an inactivated vaccine at 9 months *after* receiving HT at 5 months were significantly more likely to die from other causes compared with girls who received an inactivated vaccine at 5 months *before* receiving a standard measles vaccine at 9 months (mortality rate ratio, MRR = 1.89).

- Girls who received HT at 5 months of age did not have increased mortality until after they received inactivated vaccines at 9 months of age.

- Girls who received DTP concurrent with their 9-month measles vaccination also had significantly high mortality (MRR = 2.00). Boys did not have higher mortality regardless of when the inactivated vaccine was administered.

- This paper shows that DTP and polio vaccines can have non-specific effects that increase susceptibility to fatal diseases not targeted by the vaccine.

266.

Girls who receive a DTP vaccine simultaneously with a measles vaccine have increased morbidity and poor growth

"The present randomised trial indicates that the current practice of combining DTP...with measles vaccine had negative effects on growth and morbidity for girls."

Agergaard J, Nante E, et al. **Diphtheria-tetanus-pertussis vaccine administered simultaneously with measles vaccine is associated with increased morbidity and poor growth in girls. A randomised trial from Guinea-Bissau.** *Vaccine* 2011 Jan 10; 29(3): 487-500.

- Previous studies have shown that children who receive DTP together with a measles vaccine have higher mortality than children who receive a measles vaccine only. In this paper, scientists tested whether receiving DTP with a measles vaccine has negative non-specific effects on *morbidity* and *growth*.

- A total of 568 children from 9 to 48 months of age were randomized to receive a measles vaccine with DTP or a measles vaccine without DTP. (Both groups also received an oral polio vaccine.)

- Fever, crying, loss of appetite, and vomiting were significantly more common in the first 3 days after vaccination in the 'measles vaccine plus DTP' group compared with those who received a measles vaccine without DTP.

- Medical consultations, hospitalizations, and febrile disease with vesicular rash were more common in the 'measles vaccine plus DTP' group compared with those who received a measles vaccine without DTP.

- Girls in the 'measles vaccine plus DTP' group required medication 3.5 times more often compared with girls in the 'measles vaccine without DTP' group, and also had significantly more diarrhea than boys.

- At 9 months follow-up, girls who received a measles vaccine plus DTP were smaller in size and weighed significantly less than girls who received a measles vaccine without DTP. In low-income nations, poor growth is a reliable indicator for risk of subsequent mortality.

HPV, Chickenpox
and Shingles

In this chapter several studies on human papilloma virus (HPV), chickenpox, and shingles are summarized. The HPV vaccine increases the risk of serious autoimmune adverse events. Vaccinated females were 15 times more likely than controls to develop ovarian cancer, 10 times more likely to develop irritable bowel syndrome, and seven times more likely to develop systemic lupus erythematosus. They were also significantly more likely to develop arthritis, gastroenteritis, vasculitis, thrombocytopenia, and nervous system demyelinating conditions.

In Japan, the HPV vaccination program was halted in response to adverse event reports. Two large randomized studies found significantly more severe adverse events and deaths in the HPV-vaccinated versus placebo group. Canadian researchers found that 10% of all HPV-vaccinated people visited an emergency room within six weeks following vaccination. Another study found that some women may develop celiac disease after quadrivalent HPV vaccination.

The CDC suppressed scientific data on adverse public health effects associated with the universal chickenpox vaccination program. It published positive findings related to decreased cases of chickenpox following chickenpox vaccination but attempted to block a lead researcher from conducting objective research and publishing negative findings such as declining vaccine efficacy and higher rates of shingles. The CDC also supported the scientifically unsound practice of averaging out the incidence of shingles among two very different populations, those who caught chickenpox naturally and those who received the vaccine, masking high rates of shingles following universal chickenpox vaccination.

A meta-analysis identified 80 papers showing that the reactivation of herpes zoster (shingles) and other viruses occurs after covid vaccination.

267.

The HPV vaccine increases the risk of serious autoimmune adverse events, including ovarian damage, lupus, and irritable bowel syndrome

"The present study provides additional epidemiological evidence to support a significant association between HPV4 vaccine administration and specific serious autoimmune adverse events."

Geier DA, Geier MR. **Quadrivalent human papillomavirus vaccine and autoimmune adverse events: a case-control assessment of the vaccine adverse event reporting system (VAERS) database.** *Immunol Res* 2017 Feb; 65(1): 46-54.

- In this study, 48,852 adverse event reports in the Vaccine Adverse Event Reporting System (VAERS) database were analyzed to determine the risk of serious autoimmune adverse events in females following HPV4 vaccination.

- Females with the following serious autoimmune ailments were significantly more likely than controls to have received HPV4 vaccine: ovarian damage (OR = 14.96); irritable bowel syndrome (OR = 10.02); alopecia (OR = 8.89); systemic lupus erythematosus (OR = 7.63); rheumatoid arthritis (OR = 5.63); gastroenteritis (OR = 4.63); vasculitis (OR = 3.42); thrombocytopenia (OR = 2.18); central nervous system demyelinating conditions (OR = 1.59).

- Thrombocytopenia (39.13 %), lupus (28.57 %), and vasculitis (27.27 %) had the highest percentages of life-threatening outcomes. Rheumatoid arthritis (35.48 %), CNS demyelinating conditions (34.38 %), and lupus (25.00 %) had the highest percentages of permanent disabilities.

- Vasculitis had the shortest median onset of symptoms (3 days) and rheumatoid arthritis had the longest (37 days) following HPV4 vaccination.

- The non-autoimmune outcome of syncope (loss of consciousness) was also significantly associated with receipt of HPV4 vaccine (OR 5.34).

- Results found in this study are biologically plausible.

268.

In Japan, serious adverse reactions to the HPV vaccine are common; commercial interests drive HPV vaccine policy

"The human papillomavirus vaccine has been linked to a number of serious adverse reactions. The range of symptoms is diverse and they develop in a multi-layered manner over an extended period of time."

Beppu H, Minaguchi M, et al. **Lessons learnt in Japan from adverse reactions to the HPV vaccine: a medical ethics perspective.** *Indian J Med Ethics* 2017 Apr-Jun; 2(2): 82-88.

- This paper reviewed adverse reactions after HPV vaccination in Japan and the influence of vaccine manufacturers on healthcare policy and research.

- HPV vaccine symptoms include seizures, pain, motor and respiratory dysfunction, endocrine disorders, sleep disorders, autoimmune reactions, psychological disturbances, cognitive impairments, disorientation, and extreme fatigue.

- Eleven of 15 members of the expert advisory panel had conflicts of interest.

269.

Ozawa K, Hineno A, et al. **Suspected adverse effects after human papillomavirus vaccination: a temporal relationship between vaccine administration and the appearance of symptoms in Japan.** *Drug Saf* 2017 Dec; 40(12): 1219-29.

"Many symptoms after HPV vaccination are explainable by a combination of autonomic dysfunction, chronic regional pain syndrome, and cognitive dysfunction."

- A significant number of vaccinated girls experienced chronic headaches, prolonged fatigue, violent tremors, widespread joint and limb pain, cognitive and motor dysfunction, sleep disturbance, and menstrual abnormalities.

- In 2013, Japan terminated the compulsory HPV vaccine program. No new vaccine-related symptoms were observed during the follow-up period.

270.

Randomized studies and case series provide evidence that the HPV vaccine increases the risk of serious adverse events

"Two of the largest HPV vaccine randomized trials showed significantly more severe adverse events in the investigated vaccine arm of the study. Bivalent HPV immunization was accompanied by a statistically significant four-fold increase in the death rate."

Martínex-Lavin M, Amezcua-Guerra L. **Serious adverse events after HPV vaccination: a critical review of randomized trials and post-marketing case series.** *Clin Rheumatol* 2017 Oct; 36(10): 2169-2178.

- This paper reviewed serious adverse events after HPV vaccination, as described in pre-licensure randomized studies and post-marketing safety reports.

- Two of the largest randomized studies found significantly more severe adverse events in the group that received the HPV vaccine vs. placebo. There were 13 deaths in the vaccine group vs. 3 deaths in the control group.

- Canadian researchers found that 10% of all HPV-vaccinated people visited an emergency room within 6 weeks following vaccination. Spanish researchers classified 32% of HPV vaccine adverse events as "severe." In Japan, the HPV vaccination program was halted in response to adverse event reports.

- A meta-analysis conducted in six Asian countries found increased risks of arthralgia (RR = 1.94), myalgia (RR = 1.84), and systemic adverse events (RR = 1.33). The 9-valent shot has twice the viral and aluminum content as the 4-valent shot, and systemic adverse events occurred more frequently.

- Although randomized studies and safety reports described similar clusters of adverse events, they were labeled differently, diluting safety signals (e.g., fatigue and musculoskeletal pain vs. fibromyalgia and complex regional pain).

- Most randomized studies did not use an inert placebo in the control group; controls were injected with aluminum or an aluminum-containing vaccine. In some people, HPV viral matter and/or the aluminum adjuvant may damage the dorsal root ganglia, inducing dysautonomia and small fiber neuropathy.

271.

Some women may develop celiac disease after quadrivalent HPV vaccination

"After sensitivity analyses, the association between quadrivalent HPV vaccination and coeliac disease was the most robust. The observed association of a 56% increased risk of coeliac disease after quadrivalent HPV vaccination was strong, and the increase was strikingly similar in both risk periods after vaccination."

Hviid A, Svanström H, et al. **Human papillomavirus vaccination of adult women and risk of autoimmune and neurological diseases.** *J Intern Med* 2018 Feb; 283(2): 154-165.

- In this study of more than 3 million Danish and Swedish women 18-44 years of age, women who received at least one dose of the quadrivalent HPV vaccine (qHPV) were compared to women who did not receive the qHPV vaccine. (Few of the women received all 3 recommended doses.)

- Seven diseases with statistically significant increased risks after qHPV vaccination were identified: 1) Hashimoto's thyroiditis, 2) celiac disease, 3) localized lupus erythematosus, 4) pemphigus vulgaris, 5) Addison's disease, 6) Raynaud's disease, and 7) encephalitis, myelitis or encephalomyelitis.

- After the seven diseases with statistically significant increased risks were identified, the study authors reanalyzed the data using four criteria. All of the ailments except for celiac disease lost statistical significance.

- Vaccinated women were significantly more likely than unvaccinated women to develop celiac disease any time after vaccination: IRR = 1.56 and 1.65 for the cohort and the self-controlled case series method, respectively.

- The crude incidence rate for celiac disease in Denmark was 31.1 per 100,000 person-years in the vaccinated group and 13.9 in the unvaccinated group. The corresponding Swedish rates were 50.9 and 34.2. About half of all celiac cases after vaccination occurred within one year of the first dose.

- The main author of this paper acknowledged a potential conflict of interest for having previously received funding from two HPV vaccine manufacturers.

272.

HPV-vaccinated girls had more annual visits to the doctor after vaccination than non-vaccinated girls

"All vaccinated groups consulted the general practitioner more often than the non-vaccinated group."

Krogsgaard LW, Vestergaard CH, et al. **Health care utilization in general practice after HPV vaccination—A Danish nationwide register-based cohort study.** *PloS One* 2017 Sep 8; 12(9): e0184658.

- In Denmark, the HPV vaccination program has been challenged due to an increasing number of adverse events after receipt of the vaccine.

- The purpose of this study was to examine a potential link between HPV vaccination and adverse events by using physician consultations after vaccination as an indicator of vaccine-associated morbidity.

- This study analyzed the health records of 214,240 Danish 12-year-old girls who were: a) HPV-only vaccinated, b) MMR-only vaccinated, c) HPV and MMR vaccinated, d) non-vaccinated.

- Non-vaccinated girls had the fewest mean number of physician consultations during the entire study period (2008-2015).

- The mean number of physician consultations was highest in the group of HPV-only vaccinated girls.

- In the adjusted analysis, vaccinated girls in all three groups had higher physician consultation rates compared to the group of non-vaccinated girls.

- Physician consultation codes were disregarded when they appeared in the same week that a vaccination was given. Thus, it is likely that healthcare utilization rates among the vaccinated girls were underestimated in this study.

- Physician consultations is an imperfect measure of vaccine-associated morbidity; more severe morbidity associated with secondary care was not captured in this study, nor were potential vaccine-related fatalities.

273.

Some girls and young women may develop an autoimmune disease after HPV vaccination

"Probable side effects to HPV vaccination have symptoms and biological markers compatible with an autoimmune disease closely resembling that seen in myalgic encephalomyelitis or chronic fatigue syndrome."

Mehlsen J, Brinth L, et al. **Autoimmunity in patients reporting long-term complications after exposure to human papilloma virus vaccination.** *J Autoimmun* 2022 Dec; 133: 102921.

- In this study, 839 Danish females (mean age = 23.5 years) who experienced possible adverse reactions to HPV vaccination were compared to controls. The large cohort of young women with possible side-effects to HPV vaccination differed significantly from an age-matched HPV-vaccinated control group.

- All three marketed HPV vaccines—bivalent (HPV2), quadrivalent (HPV4), and nona-valent (HPV9)—contain an aluminum adjuvant. Yet, nearly all pre-licensure studies of HPV-vaccines used either an aluminum-containing injection or another vaccine as the control substance.

274.

Pierce JY, Vickers MJ, et al. **HPV vaccination uptake associated with HPV-related cancer incidence but not rurality in the Deep South: Does perceived risk outweigh access concerns?** *Gynecology Oncology* 2019 Jun; 154(Supplement 1): 9. (Presented at the *50th Annual Meeting of the Society of Gynecologic Oncology* 2019 March 16-19; Honolulu, HI: Abstract 13.)

- This study sought to determine which factors are associated with HPV vaccination rates in 13-17-year olds, by county, in the state of Alabama.

- Having public insurance ($r = 0.47$) and living in poverty ($r = 0.39$) were associated with higher HPV vaccination rates. Higher cervical cancer rates per county were correlated with higher HPV vaccination rates in females ($r = 0.49$) and males ($r = 0.46$).

275.

The CDC manipulated and suppressed scientific data on adverse public health effects associated with the universal chickenpox vaccination program

"Financial conflicts of interest, lack of proper controls, and poor methodology in varicella studies commissioned by the CDC often yielded improper or confounded results and conclusions, producing research based on pseudoscience that should more appropriately be relegated to a faith-based belief system rather than the realm of science."

Goldman GS. **The US universal varicella vaccination program: CDC censorship of adverse public health consequences.** *Ann Clin Pathol* 2018 Mar 31; 6(2): 1133.

- The author of this paper was hired to help monitor the effects of the CDC's new chickenpox vaccination program and conduct epidemiological studies. He resigned 8 years later in protest against scientific fraud and began exposing actions by the CDC contributing to obfuscation and malfeasance.

- The CDC published positive findings related to decreased cases of chickenpox following chickenpox vaccination but attempted to block the author from conducting objective research and publishing negative findings such as declining vaccine efficacy and higher rates of herpes zoster (shingles).

- The CDC supported the scientifically unsound practice of averaging out the incidence of shingles among two very different populations — those who caught chickenpox naturally and those who received the vaccine — masking high rates of shingles following universal varicella vaccination.

- The CDC conducted a study on shingles in a population where the varicella vaccine had not been widely distributed, providing false evidence that the varicella vaccination program did not increase shingles rates.

- The CDC made 3 false assumptions to justify universal varicella vaccination: 1) the vaccine would cost $35 per dose, 2) a single dose would provide lifelong immunity, and 3) there would be no increased cases of shingles.

276.

Japan, Germany, and Israel saw shingles rates increase when chickenpox vaccination was introduced

"Our long-term surveillance of herpes zoster clarified that universal varicella vaccination increased the incidence of herpes zoster in the child-rearing generation."

Toyama N, Shiraki K. **Universal varicella vaccination increased the incidence of herpes zoster in the child-rearing generation as its short-term effect.** *J Dermatol Sci* 2018 Oct; 92(1): 89-96.

- In Japan, universal varicella vaccination was initiated in 2014. From 2014 to 2016, as cases of chickenpox declined the incidence of herpes zoster significantly increased in adults 20 to 49 years of age (odds ratio, OR = 1.27).

277.

Diehl R, Wiedenmann C, et al. **Increasing hospitalisation of patients with herpes zoster ophthalmicus-an interdisciplinary retrospective analysis.** *Graefes Arch Clin Exp Ophthalmol* 2024 Feb; 262(2): 583-588.

"If herpes zoster ophthalmicus continues to increase, the number of hospitalisations of zoster ophthalmicus would double by 2040."

- In Germany, from 2009-2022 there was a 200% increase in HZ cases.

278.

Forer E, Yariv A, et al. **The association between varicella vaccination and herpes zoster in children: a semi-national retrospective study.** *J Clin Med* 2023 Jun 27; 12(13): 4294.

A total of 109 herpes zoster cases per 100,000 population per year were diagnosed between 2000 and 2007 (pre-vaccination era), compared to 354 herpes zoster cases per 100,000 population per year diagnosed between 2008 and 2021 (post-vaccination era) (p < 0.001).

279.

Herpes zoster and other viruses are reactivated after covid vaccination

"Our study showed the possible association between COVID-19 vaccination and herpesvirus reactivation."

Shafiee A, Amini MJ, et al. **Herpesviruses reactivation following COVID-19 vaccination: a systematic review and meta-analysis.** *Eur J Med Res* 2023 Aug 10; 28(1): 278.

- Among those who received covid vaccines, several reports have been published regarding the reactivation of herpes simplex virus, varicella-zoster virus, Epstein-Barr virus, and Cytomegalovirus.

- This systematic review identified 80 papers where herpesvirus reactivation after covid vaccination was reported.

- Among those who received the covid vaccine, the rate of varicella-zoster virus reactivation was 14 persons per 1000 vaccinations and the rate of herpes simplex reactivation occurred at a rate of 16 persons per 1000 vaccinations.

- Several covid vaccines also caused the reactivation of Epstein-Barr and Cytomegaloviruses.

280.

Triantafyllidis KK, Giannos P, et al. **Varicella zoster virus reactivation following COVID-19 vaccination: a systematic review of case reports.** *Vaccines (Basel)* 2021 Sep 11; 9(9): 1013.

"Herpes zoster is possibly a condition physicians and other healthcare professionals may expect to see in patients receiving COVID-19 vaccines."

- This systematic review identified 12 papers which included 91 patients with herpes zoster following covid vaccination.

- Symptoms developed 5.8 days after vaccination, irrespective of dose.

Rotavirus

Rotavirus is a common cause of diarrhea and vomiting in children. It occurs most often in the winter months. Symptoms typically last from 3 to 8 days and may include a fever and abdominal pain. Although babies 6 months to 2 years are most vulnerable to rotavirus infection, nearly all children are exposed to this contagious microbe at least once by the time they are 5 years old.

The illness causes partial immunity because repeat infections are less severe. In most cases, rotavirus is mild enough that parents can care for their children at home. However, in severe cases dehydration and death are possible. Over 80 percent of all rotavirus deaths occur in poor countries where babies are malnourished and there is limited access to advanced healthcare. In the United States, about 20 deaths per year are attributed to this disease.

Treatment mainly consists of preventing dehydration by giving fluids until the disease runs its course. In serious cases, frequent vomiting makes oral hydration ineffective. Babies unable to keep down liquids risk dying from dehydration and require intravenous fluids.

The scientific studies in this chapter reveal some of the risks associated with the rotavirus vaccine. Intussusception is the most serious risk. Intussusception is a life-threatening medical condition in which a portion of the intestine folds into the section immediately ahead of it. Symptoms include severe abdominal pain, vomiting, and rectal bleeding often requiring surgery.

Another concern is that children vaccinated against rotavirus can still contract the disease. Also, there are several strains of rotavirus. When wild strains of rotavirus are targeted by a vaccine, new strains emerge reducing vaccine effectiveness.

281.

The rotavirus vaccine significantly increases the risk of severe intestinal damage

"The fact that intussusception reports to VAERS clustered during days 3-8 following the first dose of Rotarix, which corresponds to the period of peak intestinal replication of vaccine virus, supports the biologic plausibility of an association."

Haber P, Parashar UD, et al. **Intussusception after monovalent rotavirus vaccine — United States, Vaccine Adverse Event Reporting System (VAERS), 2008-2014.** *Vaccine* 2015 Sep 11; 33(38): 4873-77.

- Intussusception is a life-threatening medical condition in which a portion of the intestine folds into the section immediately ahead of it. Symptoms include severe abdominal pain, vomiting, and rectal bleeding often requiring surgery. Intussusception may occur following a rotavirus vaccine.

- This study utilized the Vaccine Adverse Event Reporting System (VAERS) to compare the average daily reports of intussusception that occurred 3-6 days versus 0-2 days after rotavirus vaccination.

- Of 108 confirmed reports of intussusception after rotavirus vaccination, a significant clustering occurred on days 3-8 after the first dose ($p = 0.001$), and days 2-7 after the second dose ($p = 0.001$).

- The daily reporting ratio comparing the 3-6 day and the 0-2 day periods after the first dose of rotavirus vaccine was significantly elevated, which supports the plausibility of a true association between vaccination and intussusception.

- In a sensitivity analysis, the risk of intussusception ranged from 1.2 to 2.8 excess cases per 100,000 vaccinations. If all U.S. children are vaccinated, about 68 new cases of intussusception following the first dose would be expected annually (with an estimated range of 13 to 247 cases annually).

- Of the 108 confirmed reports of intussusception, 44% required surgery, with one death reported.

282.

FDA research confirms a significantly increased risk of intussusception following rotavirus vaccines

"In the analyses of dose 1 and of all doses of RotaTeq, the temporal scan statistic showed a significant cluster of onset of intussusception 3 to 7 days after vaccination. For all doses of Rotarix, there was a significant cluster on day 4 after vaccination."

Yih WK, Lieu TA, et al. **Intussusception risk after rotavirus vaccination in U.S. infants.** *N Engl J Med* 2014 Feb 6; 370(6): 503-12.

- In 1999, the first U.S. rotavirus vaccine, RotaShield, was withdrawn from the market after causing intussusception. Two new rotavirus vaccines, RotaTeq and Rotarix, were subsequently licensed. However, international studies have linked these vaccines to an increased risk of intussusception.

- This study was conducted to evaluate the risk of intussusception among U.S. infants following receipt of RotaTeq and Rotarix vaccines. The study population included infants enrolled in three U.S. health plans.

- The primary analysis compared the risk of intussusception 1-7 days and 1-21 days after vaccination to a control interval 22-42 days after vaccination. RotaTeq was associated with a significantly increased risk of intussusception after the first dose, with about 1.5 excess cases per 100,000 vaccinations.

- The relative risk of intussusception 1-7 days after RotaTeq vaccination was 9.1 (95% CI, 2.2 to 38.6).

- In the secondary analysis using a cohort design, Rotarix was associated with a significantly increased risk of intussusception after the second dose, with an attributable risk of 7.3 excess cases per 100,000 vaccinations.

- Significant clusters of intussusception occurred 3-7 days after RotaTeq vaccination ($p = 0.008$ for dose 1; $p = 0.004$ for all doses), and on day 4 for all doses of Rotarix vaccination ($p < 0.001$).

- This study was funded by the Food and Drug Administration (FDA).

283.

Infants have a 6- to 15-fold increased risk of intussusception after rotavirus vaccination

"Our results provide evidence that both currently licensed rotavirus vaccines are associated with a similar increase in the incidence of intussusception after the first vaccine dose, estimated at 6- to 10-fold in the first 7 days and 3- to 6-fold in the 8-21 days after vaccination."

Carlin JB, Macartney KK, et al. **Intussusception risk and disease prevention associated with rotavirus vaccines in Australia's National Immunization Program.** *Clin Infect Dis* 2013 Nov; 57(10): 1427-34.

- The authors assessed the risk of intussusception after Rotarix or RotaTeq vaccines.

- In the first analysis, the relative incidence of intussusception 1-7 days after the first dose was 6.8 ($p < 0.001$) for Rotarix and 9.9 ($p < 0.001$) for RotaTeq. The risk remained significant after the second dose and during the 8-21 day post-vaccine periods.

- In the second analysis, infants that received Rotarix had a 15-fold increased risk of intussusception 1-7 days after the first dose (odds ratio, OR = 15.6). Recipients of RotaTeq had a nearly 12-fold increase (OR = 11.7). The risk remained significant during the 8-21 day post-vaccination period.

284.

Weintraub ES, Baggs J, et al. **Risk of intussusception after monovalent rotavirus vaccination.** *N Engl J Med* 2014 Feb 6; 370(6): 513-19.

"In this prospective post-licensure study of more than 200,000 doses of monovalent rotavirus vaccine, we observed a significant increase in the rate of intussusception after vaccination, a risk that must be weighed against the benefits of preventing rotavirus-associated illness."

- In this CDC-sponsored study, the relative risk (RR) of intussusception within 7 days after receiving two doses of Rotarix, as compared with a) the background rate and b) two doses of RotaTeq, was 8.4 and 9.4, respectively.

285.

Mexico and Brazil confirm an increased risk of intussusception after rotavirus vaccination

"A temporal association between vaccination and intussusception was observed within 31 days of administration of the first dose of the attenuated human rotavirus vaccine. This effect mostly occurred during the first week after vaccination."

Velázquez FR, Colindres RE, et al. **Postmarketing surveillance of intussusception following mass introduction of the attenuated human rotavirus vaccine in Mexico.** *Pediatr Infect Dis J* 2012 Jul; 31(7): 736-44.

- This study of Mexican infants was conducted to assess a potential association between the Rotarix rotavirus vaccine and intussusception.

- The relative incidence of intussusception during three pre-defined risk periods, within 31, 16, and 7 days after the first dose of the rotavirus vaccine, was 1.75 ($p=0.001$), 3.24 ($p<0.001$), and 6.49 ($p<0.001$), respectively. Surgery was required in 90% of cases. Six infants died following surgery.

286.

Patel MM, López-Collada VR, et al. **Intussusception risk and health benefits of rotavirus vaccination in Mexico and Brazil.** *N Engl J Med* 2011 Jun 16; 364(24): 2283-92.

"A combined annual excess of 96 cases of intussusception in Mexico (approximately 1 per 51,000 infants) and in Brazil (approximately 1 per 68,000 infants) and of 5 deaths due to intussusception was attributable to the monovalent rotavirus vaccine."

- This study was designed to assess an association between the Rotarix rotavirus vaccine and intussusception in Mexico and Brazil.

- In Mexico, 3 infants died. In Brazil, 16 infants died. Surgery was required in 87% of the case patients in Mexico and in 95% of the case patients in Brazil.

287.

Extending the allowable age to vaccinate infants against rotavirus increases the risk of intussusception

"Defining the acceptable risk for a vaccination program and how to manage and mitigate such risk remains a challenge. The exact intussusception risk in Norway is yet to be determined."

Bruun T, Watle SSV, et al. **Intussusception among Norwegian children: What to expect after introduction of rotavirus vaccination?** *Vaccine* 2019 Sep 10; 37(38): 5717-23.

- Recent studies have shown that currently licensed rotavirus vaccines increase the risk of intussusception about 1-5 cases per 100,000 vaccinated infants.

- To reduce the risk of intussusception, Norway adopted strict age limits for rotavirus vaccination — the second dose cannot be given past 16 weeks of age — limiting the number of fully vaccinated infants. This study estimated the incidence of intussusception under current and extended age limits.

- In the 2019 birth cohort (~60,000), 1.2 vaccine-related intussusception cases (2/100,000) would occur under current age limits. If age limits were extended to 24 weeks for the second dose — allowing more infants to be vaccinated at a riskier age — 2.2 cases per birth cohort (3.7/100,000) would be expected.

- Vaccine-associated cases of intussusception are often measured against a pre-vaccine baseline incidence, which varies greatly by country. Differences may be due to diagnostic and reporting practices or from study protocols that include definite cases, probable cases, or all cases coded as intussusception.

- Rotavirus vaccine-associated cases of intussusception are more sensitive to an increase in the age at vaccination than increased vaccine coverage.

- Few European nations support a universal rotavirus vaccination program. France ended their program after vaccine-related intussusception deaths.

- The authors of this paper concluded that an increase in intussusception cases would be offset by the number of rotavirus cases averted by vaccination.

288.

The first rotavirus vaccine in the U.S. was discontinued after causing numerous cases of intussusception

"Illness and death may result both from wild rotavirus disease and from intussusception related to the rotavirus vaccine (RRV-TV). This study provides evidence of a causal association between RRV-TV and intussusception. The association was strong, temporal, and specific."

Murphy TV, Gargiullo PM, et al. **Intussusception among infants given an oral rotavirus vaccine.** *N Engl J Med* 2001 Feb 22; 344(8): 564-72.

- In October 1998, the first rotavirus vaccine, RotaShield, was administered to U.S. infants. By May 1999, vaccination was suspended and an investigation initiated after several cases of intussusception were reported.

- There was a significantly elevated risk of intussusception 3-7 days after the 1st and 2nd doses (IRR = 58.9 and 11.0, respectively). Up to 732 additional cases would occur annually if a national program was fully implemented.

289.

Kramarz P, France EK, et al. **Population-based study of rotavirus vaccination and intussusception.** *Pediatr Infect Dis J* 2001 Apr; 20(4): 410-16.

"RotaShield is associated with an increased risk of intussusception. The risk is greatest 3 to 7 days after the first vaccination dose."

- Shortly after the first rotavirus vaccine, RotaShield, was introduced in the U.S., preliminary data from a Phase IV post-marketing study found that the incidence rate of intussusception within one week after vaccination was 314/100,000 compared with 45/100,000 in unvaccinated infants.

- In this study, RotaShield was given to 56,253 infants. The relative risk (RR) of intussusception 3-7 days post-vaccination was 30.4 after the first dose

- The CDC terminated its recommendation for the routine use of RotaShield due to the findings in this paper and the previous one by Murphy.

290.

A "catch-up" vaccination schedule increases the risk of intussusception

"The practice of initiating immunization after age 90 days, which we call "catch-up" vaccination, contributed disproportionately to the occurrence of intussusception associated with the use of RotaShield."

Simonsen L, Viboud C, et al. **More on RotaShield and intussusception: the role of age at the time of vaccination.** *J Infect Dis* 2005 Sep 1; 192 Suppl 1: S36-43.

• This paper re-analyzed data from an earlier study (Murphy et al.) to determine whether high rates of intussusception after the first dose of RotaShield were affected by the age of the infant at the time of vaccination.

• The risk of intussusception within 21 days after the first dose of RotaShield, for babies aged 1-2 months, 3-4 months, and 5-11 months, increased with age (ORs = 5.7, 10.5, and 15.9, respectively).

• Infants who were 90 days of age or older had received only 38% of first doses but accounted for 80% of intussusception cases ($p < .0001$).

• A "catch-up" immunization schedule should be avoided by completing the first dose of vaccination by 60 days of age.

291.

Patel MM, Haber P, et al. **Intussusception and rotavirus vaccination: a review of the available evidence.** *Expert Rev Vaccines* 2009 Nov; 8(11): 1555-64.

• This paper reviewed the evidence of a link between rotavirus vaccination and intussusception, and confirmed a higher risk at 3-7 days post-RotaShield in infants who received their first dose later than recommended.

• The risk of intussusception 3-7 days after the first dose of RotaShield, for babies aged 1-2 months, 3-4 months, and 5-11 months, increased with age (ORs = 30.0, 30.7, and 55.2, respectively).

292.

Wild-type rotavirus does not cause intussusception and may be protective against it

"Wild-type rotavirus was not associated with intussusception. Future research is needed to better understand the mechanisms that lead to intussusception, particularly after rotavirus vaccination."

Burnett E, Kabir F, et al. **Infectious etiologies of intussusception among children less than 2 years old in 4 Asian countries.** *J Infect Dis* 2020 Apr 7; 221(9): 1499-1505.

- This study evaluated which infectious agents cause intussusception in children less than 2 years old in Bangladesh, Nepal, Pakistan, and Vietnam prior to the introduction of rotavirus vaccination programs.

- Wild-type rotavirus was not associated with intussusception, which previous studies concluded as well. Two studies showed a protective effect.

293.

Pérez-Ortín R, Santiso-Bellón C, et al. **Rotavirus symptomatic infection among unvaccinated and vaccinated children in Valencia, Spain.** *BMC Infect Dis* 2019 Nov 27; 19(1): 998.

"The present study has revealed symptomatic rotavirus infections among fully vaccinated children. Higher levels of vaccination among children under 3 years of age was observed; however, it was precisely this age group that experienced the greatest number of infections."

- This study investigated symptomatic rotavirus infections among vaccinated children. Thirty percent of children who were diagnosed with symptomatic rotavirus infection were previously vaccinated against rotavirus.

- Current rotavirus vaccines were made to combat strains circulating in the 1980s. Today, circulating strains have diversified due to evolutionary factors. Also, atypical rotavirus strains can arise via reassortment between a human strain and RotaTeq vaccine strains.

294.

High rotavirus vaccination rates may induce new strains to emerge reducing vaccine effectiveness

"The distribution of circulating rotavirus genotypes in Botswana changed after vaccine implementation."

Mokomane M, Esona MD, et al. **Diversity of rotavirus strains circulating in Botswana before and after introduction of the monovalent rotavirus vaccine.** *Vaccine* 2019 Oct 8; 37(43): 6324-28.

• This study compared rotavirus genotypes (strains) circulating in Botswana before and after a national rotavirus vaccine program was introduced. During the pre-vaccine period, the predominant circulating strains were G9P[8] and G1P[8]. During the vaccine period, G2P[4] became the predominant genotype.

• When common strains decline in prevalence due to vaccine pressure, other strains are likely to predominate which could cause new rotavirus epidemics, as occurred in Botswana just 6 years after the vaccine program was initiated.

295.

Maguire JE, Glasgow K, et al. **Rotavirus epidemiology and monovalent rotavirus vaccine effectiveness in Australia: 2010-2017.** *Pediatrics* 2019 Oct; 144(4): e20191024.

"Reduced vaccine effectiveness...suggests waning protection. G8 genotypes have not been common in Australia, and their emergence, along with equine-like G3P[8], may be related to vaccine-induced selective pressure."

• During the pre-vaccine period in Australia, the most common genotypes were G1P[8] and G2P[4]. In the vaccine period, different genotypes such as G3P[8] and G12P[8] emerged. By 2017, G3P[8] and G8P[8] were predominant. The median age of cases rose from 3.9 years in 2010 to 7.1 years in 2017.

• High vaccination rates might have induced selective pressure leading to the emergence of G8 and other previously uncommon strains.

Mercury and Aluminum

Several vaccines containing mercury were phased out of the childhood immunization schedule from 1999 through January 2003. They were replaced with low-mercury or "thimerosal-free" vaccines. Autism rates continued to rise in the years that followed, leading health authorities to claim that autism is not linked to mercury in vaccines and that vaccination policies are safe. (If mercury in vaccines contributed to autism, then rates should have dropped after it was removed.) However, in 2002, during this so-called phase-out period, the CDC added two doses of mercury-containing influenza vaccines urged for all babies 6 to 23 months of age. Two years later, the CDC also added pregnant women in their first trimester to the list of people officially recommended and actively encouraged to receive influenza vaccines, even though a majority of available doses contained mercury.

Aluminum adjuvants are added to many vaccines to elicit a robust immune response and increase vaccine efficacy. In the United States, Canada, Europe, Australia, and many other parts of the world, infants and young children receive high quantities of aluminum from multiple inoculations. For example, in the U.S. the hepatitis B, DTaP, pneumococcal, Hib, and hepatitis A vaccines are all given during early childhood. Each of these vaccines contains aluminum, and multiple doses are required. Infants are injected with 1,225 mcg of aluminum at 2 months, and 4,925 mcg of cumulative aluminum by age 18 months.

The studies in this chapter document deleterious effects associated with mercury and aluminum in vaccines. For example, mercury-containing vaccines increase the risk of emotional disturbances, learning disabilities, autism, tics, attention deficit hyperactivity disorder (ADHD), premature puberty, and obesity. Aluminum-containing vaccines are associated with increased risks of autism and neurological disorders. Vaccinated infants receive quantities of aluminum that greatly exceed the FDA's safety limit, and several vaccines contain significantly more aluminum than specified by vaccine manufacturers.

Note: Several important scientific papers on mercury and aluminum were summarized in the first volume of *Miller's Review of Critical Vaccine Studies.*

296.

Mercury-containing childhood vaccines increase the risk of a pervasive developmental disorder

"This study...provides compelling new epidemiological evidence supporting a significant relationship between increasing organic mercury exposure from Thimerosal-containing childhood vaccines and the subsequent risk of a pervasive developmental disorder."

Geier DA, Kern JK, et al. **A case-control study evaluating the relationship between Thimerosal-containing *Haemophilus influenzae* type b vaccine administration and the risk for a pervasive developmental disorder diagnosis in the United States.** *Biol Trace Elem Res* 2015 Feb; 163(1-2): 28-38.

• This study evaluated the quantity of mercury infants received in their first 15 months of life from thimerosal-containing *Haemophilus influenzae* type b (Hib) vaccines and the long-term risk of being medically diagnosed with pervasive developmental disorder (PDD).

• To conduct this study, researchers analyzed the CDC's Vaccine Safety Datalink (VSD) database to identify children with and without a PDD diagnosis — the cases and controls — and then compared their infant exposures to mercury from Hib vaccines.

• Children diagnosed with PDD were significantly more likely than controls to have received greater mercury exposure (75mcg vs. 25mcg) within the first 6 months of life (OR = 1.97), and greater mercury exposure (100mcg vs. 25mcg) within the first 15 months of life (OR = 3.94).

• The effects were significant for males and females. More males than females (ratio = 4.2) were diagnosed with PDD.

• The results of this study are consistent with several other studies that examined other databases and found a significant link between mercury exposure and a subsequent PDD diagnosis.

• The study protocol was approved by the CDC.

297.

Mercury-containing hepatitis B vaccines significantly increase the risk of emotional disturbances and learning disabilities

"The results show a significant relationship between mercury exposure from Thimerosal-containing childhood vaccines and the subsequent risk of an emotional disturbance diagnosis."

Geier DA, Kern JK, et al. **Thimerosal exposure and disturbance of emotions specific to childhood and adolescence: a case-control study in the Vaccine Safety Datalink database.** *Bran Inj* 2017; 31(2): 272-78.

- This study evaluated the quantity of mercury infants received in their first 6 months of life from thimerosal-containing hepatitis B vaccines and the long-term risk of being medically diagnosed with an emotional disturbance. The CDC's Vaccine Safety Datalink (VSD) database was used for this purpose.

- Children diagnosed with an emotional disturbance were significantly more likely than controls to have received greater mercury exposure within the first or second month of life (odds ratio, OR = 1.34) and first 6 months of life (OR = 2.37). The effects were significant for males but not for females.

298.

Geier DA, Kern SK, et al. **A longitudinal cohort study of the relationship between Thimerosal-containing hepatitis B vaccination and specific delays in development in the US: assessment of attributable risk and lifetime care costs.** *J Epidemiol Glob Health* 2016 Jun; 6(2): 105-18.

"[This study raises] alarming questions about the adverse health and economic impacts of recommendations to routinely administer Thimerosal-containing childhood vaccines to infants worldwide."

- Children diagnosed with a learning disability were significantly more likely than controls to have received greater mercury exposure within the first month of life (12.5mcg vs. 0mcg; RR = 1.22), first 2 months of life (25mcg vs. 0mcg; RR = 1.21), and first 6 months of life (37.5mcg vs. 0mcg; RR = 2.67).

299.

Mercury-containing childhood vaccines increase the risk of autism spectrum disorder, tic disorder, and ADHD

"The results suggest that mercury exposure from thimerosal is significantly associated with the abnormal connectivity spectrum disorders of autism spectrum disorder, tic disorder, and ADHD."

Geier DA, Kern JK, et al. **Abnormal brain connectivity spectrum disorders following Thimerosal administration: a prospective longitudinal case-control assessment of medical records in the Vaccine Safety Datalink.** *Dose-Response* 2017 March 16; 15(1): 1559325817690849.

- This study evaluated the quantity of mercury infants received in their first 15 months of life from thimerosal-containing *Haemophilus influenzae* type b (Hib) vaccines and being diagnosed with autism, tic disorder, or ADHD.

- Children diagnosed with autism (OR = 1.49 per 25mcg; 2.48 per 75mcg), tic disorder (OR = 1.43 per 25mcg; 2.28 per 75mcg), or ADHD (OR = 1.50 per 25mcg; 2.51 per 75mcg) were significantly more likely than controls to have received greater mercury exposure within the first 15 months of life.

300.

Geier DA, Kern JK, Geier MR. **Increased risk for an atypical autism diagnosis following Thimerosal-containing vaccine exposure in the United States: a prospective longitudinal case-control study in the Vaccine Safety Datalink.** *J Trace Elem Med Biol* 2017 July; 42: 18-24.

"Thimerosal is significantly associated with overall and dose-dependent increased risk for atypical autism diagnoses. It is recommended that Thimerosal should be eliminated from all vaccines."

- Children diagnosed with atypical autism were significantly more likely than controls to have received greater mercury exposure within the first month of life (odds ratio, OR = 5.01), first 2 months of life (OR = 4.87), and first 6 months of life (OR = infinity). Both genders were significantly affected.

301.

Mercury-containing childhood vaccines increase the risk of attention deficit hyperactivity disorder (ADHD) and Tourette's syndrome

"In this epidemiological study, organic mercury exposure from Thimerosal-containing vaccines was found to be a significant risk factor for a hyperkinetic syndrome of childhood diagnosis."

Geier DA, Kern JK, et al. **Thimerosal-preserved hepatitis B vaccine and hyperkinetic syndrome of childhood.** *Brain Sci* 2016 Mar 15; 6(1): 9.

- This study evaluated the quantity of mercury infants received in their first 6 months of life from thimerosal-containing hepatitis B vaccines and the long-term risk of a child being medically diagnosed with hyperkinetic syndrome of childhood (HSC), including ADHD.

- Children diagnosed with HSC were significantly more likely than controls to have received greater mercury exposure within the first month of life (12.5mcg vs. 0mcg; OR = 1.45), first 2 months of life (25mcg vs. 0mcg; OR = 1.43), and first 6 months of life (37.5mcg vs. 0mcg; OR = 4.51).

302.

Geier DA, Kern JK, et al. **Thimerosal exposure and increased risk for diagnosed tic disorder in the United States: a case-control study.** *Interdiscip Toxicol* 2015 Jun; 8(2): 68-76.

"Organic mercury exposure from Thimerosal-containing childhood vaccines was determined to be a significant risk factor for the subsequent diagnosis of tic disorder."

- Children diagnosed with tic disorder were significantly more likely than controls to have received greater mercury exposure within the first month of life (12.5mcg vs. 0mcg; OR = 1.59), first 2 months of life (25mcg vs. 0mcg; OR = 1.59), and first 6 months of life (37.5mcg vs. 0mcg; OR = 2.97).

303.

Mercury-containing childhood vaccines increase the risk of premature puberty and obesity

"This study shows a dose-dependent association between increasing organic mercury exposure from Thimerosal- containing hepatitis B vaccines administered within the first six months of life and the long-term risk of the child being diagnosed with premature puberty."

Geier DA, Kern JK, Geier MR. **Premature puberty and Thimerosal-containing hepatitis B vaccination: a case-control study in the Vaccine Safety Datalink.** *Toxics* 2018 Nov 15; 6(4): 67.

- According to the EPA, mercury accumulates in the endocrine system and can affect sex hormones. Yet, mercury is added to some vaccines which could increase the risk of developing premature puberty. In this study, children with and without premature puberty were compared.

- Children diagnosed with premature puberty were significantly more likely to have received increased doses of mercury from hepatitis B vaccines in their first month of life (OR = 1.80), first two months of life (OR = 1.77), and first six months of life (OR = 2.10), compared to control subjects.

304.

Geier DA, Kern JK, et al. **Thimerosal-containing hepatitis B vaccine exposure is highly associated with childhood obesity: a case-control study using the Vaccine Safety Datalink.** *N Am J Med Sci* 2016 Jul; 8(7): 297-306.

"It is apparent that organic mercury exposure from Thimerosal-containing childhood vaccines may be an important environmental factor in the recent rapid increase in childhood obesity in the US."

- Children diagnosed with obesity were significantly more likely than controls to have received greater mercury exposure within the first month of life (odds ratio, OR = 1.51), first 2 months of life (OR = 1.49), and first 6 months of life (OR = 3.80). The effects were highly significant for males and females.

305.

Aluminum adjuvants in vaccines may induce autism in genetically vulnerable children

"Significant quantities of aluminium introduced via immunisation could produce chronic neuropathology in genetically susceptible children. Accordingly, it is recommended that the use of aluminium salts in immunisations should be discontinued and that adults should take steps to minimise their exposure to environmental aluminium."

Morris G, Puri BK, Frye RE. **The putative role of environmental aluminium in the development of chronic neuropathology in adults and children. How strong is the evidence and what could be the mechanisms involved?** *Metab Brain Dis* 2017 Oct; 32(5): 1335-1355.

- Autism and Alzheimer's disease are increasingly considered to be caused by a combination of genetic, epigenetic, and environmental factors.

- No single gene accounts for more than 1% of autism cases. Autism rates are increasing; current estimates range from 1 in 68 (1.5%) to 1 in 38 (2.6%).

- This paper reviews extensive evidence showing that aluminum adjuvants in vaccines may induce autism in genetically susceptible people. The potential for aluminum to increase the risk of Alzheimer's disease is reviewed as well.

- Aluminum has no known beneficial physiological function in the human body. Some genetic variations can predispose certain people to its adverse effects.

- Animal and human studies show that aluminum adjuvants can induce ASIA syndrome, lupus, neurocognitive impairment, rheumatoid arthritis, and autism.

- Chronic aluminum exposure causes a reduction in glutathione with severe detrimental effects on anti-oxidant defenses. Aluminum can also induce mitochondrial dysfunction, microglial activation, astrocyte apoptosis, and pro-inflammatory cytokines, all associated with autism.

- The authors recommend avoiding unnecessary exposure to environmental sources of aluminum salts, especially children, pregnant mothers, and women of childbearing age who may become pregnant.

306.

Very high levels of aluminum in the brains of people with autism suggest a link to aluminum-containing vaccines

"We have made the first measurements of aluminium in brain tissue in autism spectrum disorder and we have shown that the brain aluminium content is extraordinarily high."

Mold M, Umar D, et al. **Aluminium in brain tissue in autism.** *J Trace Elem Med Biol* 2018 Mar; 46: 76-82.

• Several childhood vaccines contain an aluminum adjuvant and their expanded use has been directly correlated with increasing cases of autism.

• In this study, the brains of five deceased people 15-50 years old who had been diagnosed with autism were analyzed (using transversely heated graphite furnace atomic absorption spectroscopy) to determine the aluminum content in temporal, frontal, parietal, occipital, and hippocampus tissue.

• Approximately 67% of brain tissues examined had an aluminum content considered pathologically significant. The brains of all 5 people had at least one tissue with a pathologically significant quantity of aluminum.

• Aluminum-selective fluorescence microscopy was used to examine the brain tissue of 10 additional donors who were diagnosed with autism. Aluminum deposits were detected in all of their brains.

• Aluminum deposits were significantly more prevalent in males than females. In males, most of the aluminum deposits were intracellular whereas in females a majority were extracellular.

• Aluminum was found in both white and grey matter. White blood cells loaded with aluminum were identified in the meninges possibly entering brain tissue from the lymphatic system. Non-neuronal cells including inflammatory cells, glial cells and microglia were loaded with aluminum.

• Aluminum detected in inflammatory cells in the meninges, brain vasculature, white and grey matter could implicate aluminum in the etiology of autism.

307.

Mice injected with the lowest dose of a common aluminum adjuvant used in human vaccines developed the worst neurobehavioral and brain pathologies

"In the context of massive development of vaccine-based strategies worldwide, the present study may suggest that aluminium adjuvant toxicokinetics and safety require reevaluation."

Crépeaux G, Eidi H, et al. **Non-linear dose-response of aluminium hydroxide adjuvant particles: Selective low dose neurotoxicity.** *Toxicology* 2017 Jan 15; 375: 48-57.

- In this study, scientists injected mice with varying doses of an aluminum adjuvant widely used in human vaccines. Six months later, the mice were evaluated for 1) cognitive and motor functions, 2) immune activation in the brain, 3) cerebral aluminum levels, and 4) granulomas at the injection site.

- There were 4 experimental groups of 10 mice per group. The mice received 3 injections (4 days apart) of either 200, 400, or 800 mcg of Al/kg of body weight — equivalent to a human receiving 2, 4, or 8 doses of an aluminum-containing vaccine. The fourth group of mice received a placebo.

- Animals injected with aluminum at 200 mcg Al/kg had significantly decreased locomotor activity levels and less grip strength, a significant increase in the number of microglial cells in the ventral forebrain ($p = 0.03$), and significantly higher aluminum content in their brains ($p = 0.01$), compared to controls.

- Mice injected with the least amount of aluminum had the highest quantity in the brain, the most neurobehavioral changes, but virtually no granulomas (aluminum-filled lesions at the site of vaccination).

- The lowest dose of aluminum produced the worst behavioral outcomes, microglial (immune) activation, and cerebral aluminum level increases.

- This study suggests that lower doses of injected aluminum may be more neurotoxic than higher doses that form granulomas at the injection site.

308.

Aluminum adjuvants in vaccines can cause neurological disorders

"There is now sufficient evidence from a great number of studies to call for a reevaluation of the use of aluminum additives for human consumption or as immune adjuvants."

Blaylock RL. **Aluminum-induced immunoexcitotoxicity in neuro-developmental and neurodegenerative disorders.** *Current Inorganic Chemistry* 2012; 2(1): 46-53.

- Children receive a total of 5mg of aluminum from their pediatric vaccines by 2 years of age. This paper reviews the evidence linking aluminum to immunoexcitotoxicity and neurological disorders.

- Immunoexcitotoxicity refers to the way that aluminum (and other neurotoxic metals) exert their harmful influences within the central nervous system.

- Aluminum adjuvants can cause immunoexcitotoxicity by activating microglia (the brain's primary immune cells), triggering inflammatory cytokines and excitotoxins (such as glutamate), leading to neurological disorders.

- Aluminum also disrupts several energy-related enzymes, promotes brain inflammation and oxidative damage, reduces brain antioxidants such as glutathione, and alters calcium homeostasis.

- Injected aluminum from vaccines is absorbed and distributed throughout the body. Aluminum particles within neurons and glial cells could act as persistent stimuli for immunoexcitotoxicity.

- Evidence confirms that aluminum adjuvants cause cognitive degeneration affecting executive functions such as memory, attention, and planning.

- In an immature and developing brain, aluminum-induced immunoexcito-toxicity could lead to neurodevelopmental disorders such as autism and seizures. In aging brains, progressive neurodegeneration is possible, resulting in amyotrophic lateral sclerosis (ALS), Alzheimer's or Parkinson's disease.

309.

Babies receive unsafe quantities of aluminum from their childhood vaccines

"Toxic metals such as aluminum do not belong in prophylactic medications. Parents should not be compelled to permit their loved ones to receive multiple injections of toxic metals that could increase their risk of neurodevelopmental and autoimmune ailments. Safe alternatives to current disease prevention technologies are urgently needed."

Miller NZ. **Aluminum in childhood vaccines is unsafe.** *Journal of American Physicians and Surgeons* 2016 Winter; 21(4): 109-117.

- Aluminum adjuvants are added to several vaccines to stimulate the immune system and increase vaccine efficacy. Infants and young children throughout the world receive high quantities of aluminum from multiple inoculations.

- Although aluminum is environmentally abundant, it is a widely recognized neurotoxin with a long history of well-documented adverse effects.

- Infants are repeatedly injected with aluminum from several vaccines during critical periods of brain development.

- Aluminum adjuvants in vaccines have been linked to several neurological and autoimmune ailments, including multiple sclerosis, lupus, chronic fatigue, Gulf War syndrome, macrophagic myofasciitis, arthritis, and ASIA syndrome.

- Symptoms of vaccine-induced autoimmunity can take months or years to manifest, much longer than the time utilized in most vaccine safety studies.

- Some health authorities who oversee federal vaccine programs acknowledge their limited understanding of aluminum and mercury added to vaccines.

- The FDA published a study (Mitkus et al) claiming that aluminum-containing vaccines are safe, but there are major flaws in the FDA's analysis.

- Aluminum toxicity levels established by the FDA indicate that newborns and 2-month-old infants who are vaccinated by CDC guidelines may be receiving quantities of aluminum significantly higher than safety levels.

310.

Aluminum in vaccines and fluoride in drinking water are risk factors for brain inflammation and autism

"Evidence is presented that the abundance of fluoride added to the water worldwide and the widespread availability of aluminum, particularly to infants and young children through aluminum-containing vaccines, singly or together as aluminofluoride, can be potent factors in producing the condition of immunoexcitotoxicity that leads to the pathological changes seen in autism spectrum disorders. The vaccine program should be evaluated to reduce the excessive stimulation of the immature immune system and to replace aluminum adjuvants."

Strunecka A, Blaylock RL, et al. **Immunoexcitotoxicity as the central mechanism of etiopathology and treatment of autism spectrum disorders: A possible role of fluoride and aluminum.** *Surg Neurol Int* 2018 Apr 9; 9: 74.

- Excitotoxicity refers to the pathological process by which nerve cells are damaged and killed due to over-stimulation by neurotransmitters such as glutamate. Immunoexcitotoxicity (IET) describes the interaction between excitotoxicity and inflammatory mechanisms.

- This paper reviews extensive evidence indicating that the ubiquitous toxins aluminum and fluoride can trigger and exacerbate pathological processes associated with IET and induce health effects resembling symptoms of autism.

- Prolonged and repeated systematic immune activations, which can occur with pediatric vaccines containing aluminum, may cause pathological changes in the developing brain resulting in neurobehavioral disorders such as autism.

- Excessive exposure to fluoride, commonly found in drinking water, may cause neurological harm, low IQ, learning disorders, behavior problems, and autism.

- Low doses of aluminum and fluoride are synergistically toxic, amass in the brain inducing microglial activation, inflammation, and neurodegeneration.

- IET can be treated, and the symptoms of autism ameliorated.

311.

Fluoride in drinking water may interact with aluminum in vaccines to increase the risk of neurological effects, including autism

"Basic science suggests significant interaction between fluoride and aluminum, both known neurotoxins. The mix could be additive or worse — synergistic. One might be the bullet, the other the trigger."

Rowen RJ. **Fluoridation practices — a missing link in the vaccine-autism connection?** *Medical Research Archives* Feb 2017; 5(2): 1-12.

- This paper presents a working hypothesis that fluoride in drinking water could be enhancing the toxic neurological effects of aluminum adjuvants in vaccines.

- Fluoride in drinking water has been shown to enhance aluminum uptake in rat brains and subsequent neurologic impairment.

- Concurrent exposure to aluminum and fluoride, as compared to fluoride alone, has been shown to cause a greater deprivation of neuronal integrity.

- In the USA, neurodevelopmental disorder rates are higher in cities compared to the rural south where vaccination rates are high but there is less fluoridation.

- Some U.S. cities with the highest reported rates of autism, such as Chicago, Los Angeles, Pittsburgh, and San Francisco, add fluoride to their water. In California, autism cases tend to cluster in cities with fluoridated water.

- Egypt, India, and Nigeria do not fluoridate their water and have fewer reported cases of autism compared to rates in Western nations.

- Although several childhood vaccines contain aluminum, and fluoride (from any source) may enhance its toxicity, no vaccine safety studies have controlled for fluoride exposure.

- Autism rates (and all-cause morbidity/mortality) could be studied by comparing children who receive 1) fluoride/vaccines, 2) fluoride/no vaccines, 3) no fluoride/vaccines, 4) no fluoride/no vaccines.

312.

Health authorities warrant the safety of aluminum adjuvants in vaccines by citing three flawed studies

"Given their serious conceptual and methodological weaknesses, the three available toxicokinetic studies objectively constitute insufficient bases to guarantee the absolute safety of aluminum adjuvants administered at very large scale, in particular over the long term."

Masson J, Crépeaux G, et al. **Critical analysis of reference studies on the toxicokinetics of aluminum-based adjuvants.** *J Inorg Biochem* 2018 April; 181: 87-95.

• Health regulators routinely cite three studies — Flarend el al, 1997; Keith et al, 2002; and Mitkus et al, 2011 — to justify the continued use of aluminum adjuvants in vaccines despite numerous other studies with alternate findings.

• In this paper, independent scientists closely examined these three studies to determine their validity in light of recent findings on the toxicokinetics of aluminum adjuvants in vaccines.

• The Flarend et al hypothesis — that aluminum adjuvants are soluble — is false. Once injected into a tissue, clusters of adjuvant are rapidly captured by immune cells and whisked away from the dissolving effect of chelating agents in the interstitial fluid. Study design and findings are incorrect as well.

• The Keith et al paper set the aluminum safety threshold too high, had an erroneous aluminum absorption model, and failed to account for an infant's immature filtration function.

• The Mitkus et al paper made theoretical calculations on the intake and excretion of aluminum in infants but conflated safety standards for dietary and vaccine-derived aluminum. Intestinally absorbed aluminum cannot be compared with the particulate toxicity of aluminum salts injected intramuscularly.

• Since Mitkus et al only measured soluble aluminum, disregarded the bio-persistence of particulate aluminum, and overestimated safety levels by a factor of 17, the safety of aluminum adjuvants in infants cannot be guaranteed.

313.

Scientists call for a suspension of animal studies evaluating the safety of aluminum adjuvants in vaccines

"Taking advantage of the rise of anti-animal experimentation movements to claim for a global rejection of animal studies on adjuvant safety is...an unethical way of raising a proper scientific discussion."

Gherardi RK, Crépeaux G, et al. **Animal studies are mandatory to investigate the poorly understood fate and effects of aluminum adjuvants administered to billions of humans and animals worldwide.** *Autoimmun Rev* 2018 Jul; 17(7): 735-37.

- Several animal studies have linked aluminum adjuvants used in vaccines to ASIA syndrome, an autoimmune disorder. In a recent paper [Ameratunga], the authors refute the existence of the condition and call for a suspension of animal studies evaluating the safety of aluminum adjuvants.

- In this paper, the authors systematically respond to each concern raised in the Ameratunga paper, which omitted from review several animal studies documenting neurologic effects of aluminum adjuvants.

- The aluminum adjuvant used in the HPV vaccine is proprietary to the manufacturer (not available for independent safety studies), which is unethical because it was used in pre-market trials of the vaccine and placebo.

- It is unethical for Ameratunga to suggest that animals are being tortured as a pretext to forbid animal studies evaluating the safety of aluminum adjuvants, which are used in 60% of current vaccines given to billions of people globally.

- The Institute of Medicine recently affirmed scientists' inadequate understanding of biologic mechanisms underlying vaccine adverse effects, an argument favoring continued animal studies on aluminum adjuvant safety.

- Ameratunga is an immunology specialist who prescribes aluminum-containing injections. He was paid by the government to review the existence of ASIA.

314.

Mice that were injected with an aluminum adjuvant commonly used in childhood vaccines became socially impaired, a distinctive feature of autism

"This is the first experimental study, to our knowledge, to demonstrate that aluminum adjuvants can impair social behaviour if applied in the early period of postnatal development."

Sheth SKS, Li Y, Shaw CA. **Is exposure to aluminium adjuvants associated with social impairments in mice? A pilot study.** *J Inorg Biochem* 2018 Apr; 181: 96-103.

- This study investigated the effect of aluminum adjuvants on social behavior in mice. Deficits in social behavior are a distinctive feature of autism.

- In this study, 28 mice were injected with aluminum hydroxide (a common adjuvant used in childhood vaccines) in doses adjusted to the U.S. pediatric immunization schedule. Twenty-three control mice were injected with saline. All of the mice were then tested for anomalies in social interaction.

- The aluminum-injected mice showed significantly decreased sociability compared to controls at week 8 ($p = 0.016$) and week 17 ($p = 0.012$). They also showed abnormal social novelty and memory at week 8 ($p = 0.002$) and week 29 ($p = 0.042$).

- The aluminum-injected mice also weighed significantly less over time than controls ($p = 0.001$).

- Aluminum has no known function in any biological processes and is non-essential for life. Numerous studies have linked it with neurological and immunological disorders, including Alzheimer's disease and ASIA syndrome.

- The toxic potential of aluminum is affected by the route of administration. Ingested aluminum is almost completely excreted by the kidneys. In contrast, almost 100% of injected aluminum travels to different sites in the body, such as the brain, joints, and spleen where it accumulates and is retained for years.

315.

Vaccinated infants receive quantities of aluminum that greatly exceed the FDA's safety limit

"Our calculations show that the levels of aluminum suggested by the currently used limits place infants at risk of acute, repeated, and possibly chronic exposures of toxic levels of aluminum in modern vaccine schedules."

Lyons-Weiler J, Ricketson R. **Reconsideration of the immunotherapeutic pediatric safe dose levels of aluminum.** *J Trace Elem Med Biol* 2018 Jul; 48: 67-73.

- This paper reveals several problems with prior evaluations regarding safe levels of aluminum in vaccines and provides an update on infant exposure to pediatric vaccines utilizing body weight as an assessment factor.

- The authors found two errors by the World Health Organization which led to an overestimation of safe aluminum intake levels.

- The FDA permits vaccines to contain 850 micrograms (mcg) of aluminum per dose. However, infants who receive 850 mcg of injected aluminum are exposed to levels that greatly exceed the FDA's safety limit of 4-5 mcg per kilogram (kg) of body weight per day.

- A male infant vaccinated against hepatitis B at birth receives 1800% more aluminum per body weight than a 60 kg male adult. A female infant, with lower body weight, receives an even higher burden of aluminum.

- Vaccinated infants also receive high quantities of aluminum at 2, 4, and 6 months of age.

- The maximum quantity of aluminum allowed in vaccines is based on its capacity to produce antibodies, not safety science.

- Excess exposures to aluminum in neonatal and low birthweight infants is especially concerning. Vaccination practices in the Neonatal Intensive Care Unit (NICU) must be reconsidered.

316.

Several vaccines contain significantly more aluminum than specified by vaccine manufacturers

"The aluminum content of individual vaccines within vaccine lots vary significantly. The amount of aluminum an infant receives in a vaccine is, it would appear, akin to a lottery."

Shardlow E, Linhart C, et al. **The measurement and full statistical analysis including Bayesian methods of the aluminium content of infant vaccines.** *J Trace Elem Med Biol* 2021 Jul; 66: 126762.

• Several infant vaccines contain aluminum adjuvants. Although vaccine manufacturers list the aluminum content in their patient information inserts, regulatory agencies such as the FDA and European Medicines Agency (EMA) do not independently verify the actual aluminum content.

• The aluminum content of a vaccine is measured using an unspecified method and this "proprietary information" is not made publicly available.

• In this study, independent scientists measured the aluminum content of 13 pediatric vaccines (up to 20 doses each) and compared their findings to the official amounts stated by each manufacturer on their product inserts.

• Six of the 13 vaccines (46.2%) contained significantly more aluminum than stated. Four of the 13 vaccines (30.8%) contained significantly less aluminum. Aluminum is neurotoxic, so higher quantities could be particularly unsafe. Less aluminum than recommended could affect the vaccine's efficacy.

• There is a 92% chance that the actual aluminum content of Boostrix will exceed the officially-stated quantity despite there being no statistical difference between the actual and stated quantities.

• Aluminum content is extremely variable. For example, an infant receiving Havrix could receive between 0.172 mg and 0.602 mg of aluminum per dose.

• Vaccine manufacturers and regulatory agencies must provide clarity and transparency regarding aluminum content in vaccines.

Narcolepsy and Depression

Narcolepsy is a disabling, chronic sleep disorder characterized by extreme daytime sleepiness, sleep-related hallucinations, sleep paralysis, and cataplexy (a temporary paralytic or hypnotic state). In European nations where the Pandemrix H1N1 influenza vaccine was used, the risk of developing narcolepsy was 14 to 25 times greater in children who received it than in unvaccinated children. Psychiatric disorders are common in children who developed narcolepsy after H1N1 influenza vaccine.

Vaccines have also shown a link to adolescent depression and anxiety. Major depressive disorders are commonly observed in many illnesses associated with chronic inflammation. Vaccine-induced immune stimulation can cause both acute and prolonged inflammation leading to depressive moods.

317.

The swine flu vaccine most widely used in Europe significantly increased the risk of developing narcolepsy

"Several studies from different countries using alternative methods have confirmed the association between narcolepsy and Pandemrix vaccination."

Sarkanen T, Alakuijala A, et al. **Narcolepsy associated with Pandemrix vaccine.** *Curr Neurol Neurosci Rep* 2018 Jun 1; 18(7): 43.

- During the most recent H1N1 flu pandemic, Pandemrix was the most widely used vaccine in Europe. After the vaccination campaign, the risk of narcolepsy increased 5- to 14-fold in children and adolescents, and 2- to 7-fold in adults.

- Narcolepsy is a sleep disorder characterized by excessive sleepiness and a disturbed sleep pattern. Cataplexy (sudden loss of muscle tone triggered by emotions) is a common symptom. Hypnagogic hallucinations and severe psychiatric symptoms are possible as well.

- Narcolepsy is normally a rare disease. However, the number of type 1 cases significantly increased in nations where the Pandemrix vaccine was used.

- Eight different pandemic vaccines were used in Europe. Five of these vaccines had no adjuvant. Two vaccines included MF59 as an adjuvant. Only one vaccine, Pandemrix, used AS03 as an adjuvant.

- There is increasing evidence that narcolepsy is an autoimmune disease caused by the destruction of hypocretin-producing neurons leading to hypocretin deficiency in the central nervous system. Also, narcoleptic patients had a higher immune response against the H1N1 virus than healthy controls.

- All Pandemrix-associated narcolepsy cases had predisposing genetic factors.

- Epidemiological studies indicate that an increased risk of narcolepsy occurs for up to two years after Pandemrix vaccination. The median time from vaccination to onset of narcolepsy was 42 days.

318.

The Pandemrix influenza vaccine greatly increased the risk of narcolepsy in adults

"Our study shows that the causal association between narcolepsy and the oil-in-water adjuvanted pandemic H1N1 influenza vaccine is not, as previously thought, confined to children and adolescents. We found a significantly increased risk of narcolepsy in adults following Pandemrix vaccination in England."

Stowe J, Andrews N, et al. **Risk of narcolepsy after AS03 adjuvanted pandemic A/H1N1 2009 influenza vaccine in adults: a case-coverage study in England.** *Sleep* 2016 May 1; 39(5): 1051-7.

- Narcolepsy is a disabling, chronic sleep disorder characterized by inordinate daytime sleepiness, hypnagogic hallucinations, sleep paralysis, and cataplexy.

- Previous studies showed that the Pandemrix influenza vaccine significantly increased the risk of narcolepsy in children and teens. This study investigated whether Pandemrix increased the risk of narcolepsy in adults.

- The primary analysis showed that adults with narcolepsy were 9 times more likely to have been vaccinated compared to the general population (odds ratio, OR = 9.06). The risk of narcolepsy was significantly higher when only cases with onset within 6 months of vaccination were included (OR = 17.94).

- A variation (allele) of the HLA-DQB1 gene called HLA-DQB1*06:02 is present in 95% of narcoleptic patients with cataplexy. Although a genetic predisposition plays a role in the etiology of narcolepsy, this is insufficient for the disease to develop. Environmental triggers seem to be necessary.

- Pandemrix may induce auto-antibodies to cells that produce hypocretin (orexin). Loss of these cells can cause narcolepsy with cataplexy. Alternately, antibodies to the H1N1 nucleoprotein of the Pandemrix strain may cross-react with hypocretin receptors, leading to vaccine-induced narcolepsy.

- Further research is required to understand the likely autoimmune pathway by which the oil-in-water adjuvant (AS03) and/or the viral antigens in the H1N1 Pandemrix vaccine trigger the loss of orexin-producing neurons.

319.

Norwegian children and teens developed narcolepsy after influenza vaccination

"Our results showed a marked clustering of new cases of childhood narcolepsy in the first 6 months after Pandemrix vaccination."

Heier MS, Gautvik KM, et al. **Incidence of narcolepsy in Norwegian children and adolescents after vaccination against H1N1 influenza A**. *Sleep Med* 2013 Sep; 14(9): 867-71.

- Studies in Finland and Sweden showed a sudden increase in narcolepsy cases after receipt of the Pandemrix influenza vaccine. In this study, researchers assessed a possible link between Pandemrix and narcolepsy in Norway.

- Fifty-eight children and adolescents 4-19 years of age who developed narcolepsy after receiving the Pandemrix influenza vaccine were evaluated. All of the children had excessive daytime sleepiness; 46 developed cataplexy.

- Cerebrospinal fluid hypocretin levels were measured in 41 patients, with deficiencies in all. (Loss of hypocretin-producing neurons in the hypothalamus is known to cause the symptoms of narcolepsy with cataplexy.)

- Of 37 patients analyzed, all had type HLA-DQB1*0602 — a known genetic marker indicating predisposition to narcolepsy with cataplexy.

- Data collected during 3 years following vaccination showed a significantly higher risk for narcolepsy with cataplexy, with a minimum of 10 cases per 100,000 vaccinated individuals in the first year post-vaccination ($p < .0001$).

- Some of the children had frightening hypnagogic hallucinations — including nightmares. A few developed behavioral changes with increased irritability, quarrelsomeness, and aggression. Mild depression was reported as well. Weight gain occurred in 35% of the vaccinated children with narcolepsy.

- Increased rates of narcolepsy have only been reported in nations that used the AS03 adjuvant vaccine, Pandemrix. The AS03 adjuvant contained α-tocopherol, polysorbate 80, and squalene in an oil-in-water emulsion to induce a more robust immune response to the vaccine.

320.

French children and adults developed narcolepsy after influenza vaccination

"H1N1 vaccination was strongly associated with an increased risk of narcolepsy-cataplexy in both children and adults in France."

Dauvilliers Y, Arnulf I, et al. **Increased risk of narcolepsy in children and adults after pandemic H1N1 vaccination in France.** *Brain* 2013 Aug; 136(Pt 8): 2486-96.

- From October 2009 to February 2010, France implemented a nationwide vaccination campaign against H1N1 influenza. Most vaccine recipients received Pandemrix, which contained the AS03 adjuvant (with squalene and alpha-tocopherol). Shortly thereafter, cases of narcolepsy were reported.

- In this study, French scientists investigated a link between H1N1 influenza vaccination and narcolepsy with cataplexy in children and adults in France.

- Significantly, 52.5% of narcolepsy-cataplexy cases had received H1N1 influenza vaccination prior to onset of initial symptoms versus 17.8% of their matched control subjects ($p < 10^{-4}$).

- When statistical analyses utilized the *date of diagnosis,* H1N1 vaccination increased the risk of narcolepsy-cataplexy 6-fold in children less than 18 years of age (odds ratio, OR = 6.5), and nearly 5-fold in adults (OR = 4.7).

- When statistical analyses utilized the *date of onset of initial symptoms,* H1N1 vaccination increased the risk of narcolepsy-cataplexy 27-fold in children less than 18 years of age (OR = 27.3), and 17-fold in adults (OR = 16.8).

- Median delay between vaccination and onset of initial symptoms was 2.5 months, and with diagnosis 10.6 months. However, a narcolepsy diagnosis can take up to 10 years so additional cases may remain to be identified.

- A sensitivity analysis focusing on exposure to the AS03-adjuvanted vaccine showed a significant link with narcolepsy-cataplexy in children and adults. However, "the possibility that other H1N1 vaccines may be associated with an increased risk of narcolepsy-cataplexy cannot be ruled out."

321.

Swedish children who received an H1N1 influenza vaccine were 25 times more likely than unvaccinated children to develop narcolepsy

"Pandemrix vaccination is a precipitating factor for narcolepsy, especially in combination with HLA-DQB1*0602 [a genetic marker]. The incidence of narcolepsy was 25 times higher after the vaccination compared with the time period before."

Szakács A, Darin N, Hallböök T. **Increased childhood incidence of narcolepsy in western Sweden after H1N1 influenza vaccination.** *Neurology* 2013 Apr 2; 80(14): 1315-21.

- Shortly after Sweden initiated an H1N1 influenza vaccination campaign, there were reports that narcolepsy could be a side effect of this vaccine.

- This study was conducted to assess the incidence of narcolepsy in children in western Sweden and its link to the Pandemrix H1N1 influenza vaccine.

- Scientists identified 37 children with narcolepsy; 28 had onset of symptoms post-vaccination while 9 had onset of symptoms prior to H1N1 vaccination. Symptoms included cataplexy, disturbed sleep, hallucinations, weight gain, depression with suicidal thoughts, attention deficit, and behavioral problems.

- From January 2000-August 2009 (pre-vaccination), the annual incidence of narcolepsy in children was 0.26 per 100,000, which increased to 6.6 per 100,000 during the post-vaccination period — a 25-fold increase.

- Children in the post-vaccination group had a lower age of onset — 10 years was the median age — and a more sudden onset. Two-thirds (68%) of the children in the post-vaccination group had onset of symptoms within 12 weeks; 39% developed symptoms within 6 weeks.

- The region of study (western Sweden) represents about 20% of the Swedish population, so the number of cases identified in this study would have been approximately one-fifth of those of the entire nation.

322.

In Finland, the incidence of childhood narcolepsy increased 17-fold after H1N1 influenza vaccination

"A sudden increase in the incidence of abrupt childhood narcolepsy was observed in Finland in 2010. We consider it likely that Pandemrix vaccination contributed, perhaps together with other environmental factors, to this increase in genetically susceptible children."

Partinen M, Saarenpää-Heikkilä O, et al. **Increased incidence and clinical picture of childhood narcolepsy following the 2009 H1N1 pandemic vaccination campaign in Finland.** *PLoS One* 2012; 7(3): e33723.

- Shortly after Finland initiated an H1N1 influenza vaccination campaign, numerous children developed excessive daytime sleepiness and cataplexy.

- This study was conducted to analyze the incidence of narcolepsy in Finland prior to and following the H1N1 vaccination campaign.

- From 2002-2009 (prior to the vaccination campaign), the average annual incidence of narcolepsy in children under 17 years of age was 0.31 per 100,000. In 2010, there were 5.3 cases per 100,000 — a 17-fold increase.

- From 2002-2009, the average annual incidence of narcolepsy in children under 11 years of age was 0.02 per 100,000. In 2010, there were 3.39 cases per 100,000 — a 177-fold increase.

- Fifty of 54 children had received the H1N1 influenza vaccine (Pandemrix) prior to onset of symptoms. None of the 50 children had a prior history of excessive daytime sleepiness, cataplexy, or other symptoms of narcolepsy.

- The mean age at the time of vaccination was 10.9 years and the mean age at onset of symptoms was 11.1 years.

- Nearly half (48%) of the children developed behavioral or psychiatric problems, including conduct disorder, aggressive behavior, and self-mutilation. Four of the children required psychiatric hospitalization and one patient needed antipsychotic treatment.

323.

In Ireland and England, narcolepsy in children and teens increased 14- to 18-fold after H1N1 influenza vaccination

"Our study found a significant, 13.9-fold higher risk of narcolepsy in children/adolescents vaccinated in Ireland with Pandemrix compared with unvaccinated children/adolescents."

O'Flanagan D, Barret AS, et al. **Investigation of an association between onset of narcolepsy and vaccination with pandemic influenza vaccine, Ireland April 2009-December 2010.** *Euro Surveill* 2014 May 1; 19(17): 15-25.

- This study was conducted to compare the incidence of narcolepsy in H1N1-vaccinated and unvaccinated children and adults in Ireland.

- In the primary analysis of children and teens 5-19 years of age, the incidence of narcolepsy was 0.4 per 100,000 person years in the unvaccinated group and 5.7 per 100,000 person years in the vaccinated group — a 14-fold increase (relative risk, RR = 13.9). In vaccinated adults, the RR = 20.4.

324.

Miller E, Andrews N, et al. **Risk of narcolepsy in children and young people receiving AS03 adjuvanted pandemic A/H1N1 2009 influenza vaccine: retrospective analysis.** *BMJ* 2013 Feb 26; 346: f794.

"This study shows a significantly increased risk of narcolepsy in children who received the AS03 adjuvanted pandemic strain vaccine."

- This study assessed the risk of narcolepsy in children and teens 4-18 years of age in England who received the Pandemrix vaccine.

- In a case coverage statistical analysis, children and teens who were diagnosed with narcolepsy were 18 times more likely than age-matched controls to have received an H1N1 influenza vaccine within 12 weeks prior to the onset of initial symptoms (odds ratio, OR = 18.4).

325.

In Germany, there was a 15-fold increased risk for developing narcolepsy after H1N1 influenza vaccination

"Compared with the pre-pandemic background incidence rates, the numbers of incident cases of narcolepsy within 4 and 6 months following immunization with Pandemrix were higher than expected."

Oberle D, Pavel J, Keller-Stanislawski B. **Spontaneous reporting of suspected narcolepsy after vaccination against pandemic influenza A (H1N1) in Germany.** *Pharmacoepidemiol Drug Saf* 2017 Nov; 26(11): 1321-27.

• This study investigated whether the number of confirmed narcolepsy cases in Germany following influenza vaccination with Pandemrix was higher than expected compared with the pre-vaccination background incidence rates.

• In children and adolescents 7-17 years of age at the time of symptoms onset, there was a 15-fold increased 'observed versus expected' estimate for developing narcolepsy within 4 months following vaccination ($p < 0.00001$).

• In adults 18-49 years of age, there was a 2.1-fold increased 'observed versus expected' estimate for developing narcolepsy within 4 months ($p = 0.005$).

326.

Oberle D, Drechsel-Bäuerle U, et al. **Incidence of Narcolepsy in Germany.** *Sleep* 2015 Oct 1; 38(10): 1619-28.

• This German study investigated narcolepsy rates pre- and post-pandemic.

• In children 0-9 years, the narcolepsy incidence rate significantly increased from pre-pandemic to post-pandemic (incidence density ratio, IDR = 5.00).

• In children and teens 10-17 years, the narcolepsy incidence rate significantly increased from 0.26 per 100,000 person years in the pre-pandemic period to 0.91 in the post-pandemic period (IDR = 3.50).

327.

Psychiatric disorders are prevalent in H1N1-vaccinated narcolepsy patients

"In the post-H1N1 vaccination narcolepsy group, 43% of patients had psychiatric comorbidity."

Szakács A, Hallböök T, et al. **Psychiatric comorbidity and cognitive profile in children with narcolepsy with or without association to the H1N1 influenza vaccination.** *Sleep* 2015 Apr 1; 38(4): 615-21.

• This study was conducted to evaluate psychiatric comorbidity in children who developed narcolepsy following H1N1 influenza vaccination and in children who developed narcolepsy without an association to the vaccine.

• In the group that developed narcolepsy after H1N1 vaccination, 43% had psychiatric comorbidity: 29% had attention deficit hyperactivity disorder, 20% had major depression, 10% had anxiety disorder, 7% had oppositional defiant disorder, 3% had atypical autism, and 3% had an eating disorder.

• The most common psychiatric symptom was temper tantrums, which occurred in 94% of all children who developed narcolepsy after H1N1 vaccination. They also had a significantly lower IQ, and some of the narcolepsy patients experienced daytime hallucinations.

328.

Nordstrand S, Hansen BH, et al. **Psychiatric symptoms in patients with post-H1N1 narcolepsy type 1 in Norway.** *Sleep* 2019 Apr 1;42(4): zsz008.

"The main finding from the current study of H1N1-vaccinated narcolepsy (type 1) patients was a high prevalence of internalizing psychiatric problems."

• This study found a high prevalence of psychiatric symptoms in H1N1-vaccinated narcolepsy patients. For example, 32.5% of the children had thought problems, while 27.8% of adults had attention problems. Previous studies have shown a high prevalence of ADHD in children and adults.

329.

Adolescent depression and anxiety are associated with vaccine immune responses

"What these findings suggest is the need for integrating clinical work with depressed and anxious children in a broader health context, and for considering what role immune factors may have in developmental trajectories of neurodevelopment and affective symptoms."

O'Connor TG, Moynihan JA, et al. **Depressive symptoms and immune response to meningococcal conjugate vaccine in early adolescence.** *Dev Psychopathol* 2014 Nov; 26(4 Pt 2): 1567-76.

- Previous studies have documented bi-directional interrelationships between psychological processes, the nervous system, and immune responses.

- In this study, scientists explored a link between depressive moods in 11-year-old children and immune responses to meningococcal vaccination.

- Scientists had 126 children complete psychological tests that self-assessed their degree of depression and anxiety. Pre-vaccination blood samples were collected. The children then received a quadrivalent meningococcal vaccine.

- Post-vaccination blood samples collected at 4 weeks, 3 months, and 6 months post-vaccination showed that depression and anxiety were reliably associated with higher antibody levels for serogroups W135 and Y, respectively. (The quadrivalent vaccine contains four serotypes.)

- Children with antibody concentrations above the threshold for serogroup W135 had higher levels of depression while children with immune responses above the threshold for serogroup Y had consistently higher levels of anxiety.

- In this paper, children's self-reports of mood predicted a more pronounced immune response. The effects were consistent across time and not confounded by sociodemographic or alternate health variables.

- There is growing evidence of links between immune factors and psychological or psychiatric symptoms in children. Mood disorders such as depression may lead to a pro-inflammatory state (and the reverse may be true as well).

330.

Vaccine-induced immune stimulation is associated with depressed mood

"Results confirm that the mild transient inflammatory state induced by typhoid vaccination has negative mood effects. Vaccination may be a useful model for understanding the effects of inflammation on psychological well-being."

Wright CE, Strike PC, et al. **Acute inflammation and negative mood: mediation by cytokine activation.** *Brain Behav Immun* 2005 Jul; 19(4): 345-50.

- Infectious diseases induce the production of pro-inflammatory cytokines (proteins that regulate immunity and communicate between cells). Elevated cytokine levels are associated with depression.

- In this study, scientists assessed whether the induction of acute inflammation through vaccination would increase cytokine levels and alter mood.

- Thirty healthy men took a moods test (to measure depression, anxiety, and fatigue). A baseline blood sample was drawn to measure cytokine levels. The subjects were then randomized to receive a typhoid vaccine or placebo.

- Mood scores were reassessed at 1.5, 3, and 6 hours post-vaccination. A post-vaccination blood sample was drawn at 3 hours.

- In the vaccine group, cytokine blood levels for interleuken-6 (IL-6) doubled between baseline and 3 hours post-injection (but fell in the placebo group).

- The vaccine group had a significant decline in mood between 1.5 and 3 hours post-injection. Mood levels in the vaccine group continued to drop until 6 hours post-injection. Negative mood scores at 3 hours post-injection were significantly higher in the vaccine group than in the placebo group.

- Vaccine-induced changes in IL-6 blood concentrations at 3 hours post-injection were significantly and negatively correlated with altered psychological well-being. Subjects with the greatest increases in IL-6 had the most depressed moods.

331.

Depression can result from vaccine-related activation of the immune system

"We demonstrated that, compared to control group subjects and to their own baseline, a subgroup of vulnerable individuals (girls from low socioeconomic status) showed a significant virus-induced increase in depressed mood up to 10 weeks after vaccination."

Yirmiya R, Pollak Y, et al. **Illness, cytokines, and depression.** *Ann NY Acad Sci* 2000; 917: 478-87.

• Findings in this paper provide evidence that depression can result from vaccine-related activation of the immune system.

• A significant increase in depressed mood lasting up to 10 weeks was induced in a subset of teenage girls who received a live attenuated rubella vaccine.

332.

Moreau M, André C, et al. **Inoculation of Bacillus Calmette-Guerin to mice induces an acute episode of sickness behavior followed by chronic depressive-like behavior.** *Brain Behav Immun* 2008 Oct; 22(7):1087-95.

"BCG inoculation induced an acute episode of sickness (approximately 5 days) that was followed by development of delayed depressive-like behaviors lasting over several weeks."

• This study was designed to investigate the neurological basis of depressive behavior induced by chronic inflammation after injecting mice with the BCG (*Bacillus Calmette-Guerin*) vaccine.

• This study correctly hypothesized that the initial macrophage activation by BCG vaccination would be associated with a transient episode of sickness followed by a more extensive period of depressive-like behavior.

• BCG vaccination of mice is a reliable method of inducing inflammation and depressive-like behaviors providing new data regarding the neurobiological basis through which cytokines may impact affective behaviors.

333.

Depression can be induced through vaccination and improved with phospholipid supplementation

"We suggest that phosphatidylcholine supplementation may serve as a treatment for patients suffering vaccine-related neurological manifestations."

Kivity S, Arango M, et al. **Phospholipid supplementation can attenuate vaccine-induced depressive-like behavior in mice.** *Immunol Res* 2017 Feb; 65(1): 99-105.

- Several reports have linked the human papillomavirus (HPV) vaccine with immune-mediated reactions, including neurological debilities.

- In this study, scientists evaluated the effect of a phospholipid dietary supplement on vaccine-induced depression.

- Sixty female mice were vaccinated with either an HPV/Gardasil vaccine, aluminum, or placebo. Half of the mice in each group were fed a dietary supplement enriched with phosphatidylcholine (fatty acids and phosphorous).

- Six weeks after injection, when the mice were 3 months of age, they were assessed for depression (using common and reliable tests). The HPV-vaccinated and aluminum-treated mice developed depressive-like behavior when compared to the control group.

- Multivariate regression analysis demonstrated a significant linear trend for the testing of depressive-like behavior (not attributed to motor dysfunction), indicating that mice in the Gardasil group were depressed the most, followed by mice in the aluminum group.

- Both the Gardasil and aluminum-treated mice that were fed phosphatidyl-choline showed a significant reduction in their depressive-like behavior.

- This study confirms that depressive-like behavior can be induced in mice by vaccinating them with Gardasil, and that the depressive-like behavior can be attenuated with a phosphatidylcholine-enriched diet.

Arthritis

Arthritis (pain and inflammation of the joints) has been linked to the rubella portion of the MMR vaccine, the hepatitis B vaccine, and the covid vaccine. Up to 14% of young women develop arthritis within six weeks after receiving an MMR vaccine. Girls were significantly more likely to develop joint and limb symptoms within six weeks following MMR vaccination when compared with girls who did not receive the rubella-containing shot. MMR-vaccinated children under five years of age were 12 times more likely to develop joint and limb symptoms for the first time ever when compared with children under five who did not receive MMR. Although joint and limb symptoms after MMR occurred most often in girls, the most severe cases of arthritis were in older boys.

334.

The U.S. Institute of Medicine and the National Vaccine Injury Compensation Program recognize that the rubella vaccine causes chronic arthritis

"The evidence is consistent with a causal relation between the currently used rubella vaccine strain (RA 27/3) and chronic arthritis in adult women."

Adverse Effects of Pertussis and Rubella Vaccines: A Report of the Committee to Review the Adverse Consequences of Pertussis and Rubella Vaccines. Institute of Medicine (US) Committee to Review the Adverse Consequences of Pertussis and Rubella Vaccine. Washington (DC): National Academies Press (US); 1991.

• Scientists with the U.S. Institute of Medicine found a causal link between the rubella vaccine strain (RA 27/3) and acute arthritis. Rates average 13 to 15 percent among adult women, with lower levels among children and men.

• They also found evidence of a causal link between the rubella vaccine and chronic arthritis in adult women.

• There is a biologically plausible link because the rubella virus can be found in the peripheral blood and synovial fluid of women with chronic arthritis following rubella vaccination.

335.

Weibel RE, Benor DE. **Chronic arthropathy and musculoskeletal symptoms associated with rubella vaccines. A review of 124 claims submitted to the National Vaccine Injury Compensation Program.** *Arthritis Rheum* 1996 Sep; 39(9): 1529-34.

"The National Vaccine Injury Compensation Program and the U.S. Court of Federal Claims have accepted a causal relationship between currently used rubella vaccine in the U.S. and some chronic arthropathy with onset between 1 week and 6 weeks after vaccine administration."

336.

The rubella vaccine statistically increases the risk of arthritic adverse reactions

"Our data confirms and extends the data studied by the Institute of Medicine that rubella vaccine was associated with a large number of arthritic adverse reactions. These reactions primarily occurred in the adult female population."

Geier DA, Geier MR. **Rubella vaccine and arthritic adverse reactions: an analysis of the Vaccine Adverse Events Reporting System (VAERS) database from 1991 through 1998.** *Clin Exp Rheumatol* 2001 Nov-Dec; 19(6): 724-26.

- In this study, researchers analyzed the VAERS database to determine the frequency of arthritic adverse reactions after rubella vaccination compared to the background rate of arthritic conditions in the U.S. adult population.

- Arthritic reactions were more frequent in rubella vaccine recipients compared with the control group ($p < 0.01$). For every million people vaccinated, there were 122.8 cases of arthritic reactions in excess of the background rate. Females were 12 times more likely than males to develop arthritic reactions.

- The average onset for all types of arthritic reactions was about 11 days after vaccination (with a range of 10 days to 4 weeks).

337.

Wang B, Shao X, et al. **Vaccinations and risk of systemic lupus erythematosus and rheumatoid arthritis: A systematic review and meta-analysis.** *Autoimmun Rev* 2017 July; 16(7): 756-65.

"This study suggests that vaccinations are related to increased risks of systemic lupus erythematosus and rheumatoid arthritis. More and larger observational studies are needed to further verify the findings."

- A meta-analysis of studies reporting outcomes shortly after vaccination confirms that vaccines significantly increase the risk of developing lupus (relative risk, RR = 1.93) and rheumatoid arthritis (RR = 1.48).

338.

The MMR vaccine significantly increases the risk of arthritis and arthralgia in children

"We found that exposure to measles, mumps, and rubella vaccine (MMR) was associated with an increased risk of developing joint and limb complaints in the six weeks after immunisation. The increase in risk was greater when only arthralgia or arthritis were considered. Children under 5 years were most at risk, and girls had a higher rate of first ever episodes than boys."

Benjamin CM, Chew GC, Silman AJ. **Joint and limb symptoms in children after immunisation with measles, mumps, and rubella vaccine.** *BMJ* 1992 Apr 25; 304(6834): 1075-78.

- Arthritis (pain and inflammation of the joints) has been known to occur in up to 14% of young women within 6 weeks after receiving an MMR vaccine, while up to 41% may develop arthralgia (joint pain without swelling) after MMR. However, there are limited data on the risks in children.

- In this study, researchers compared the incidence of joint and limb symptoms in 1,588 children during the 6 weeks after receiving an MMR vaccine with 1,242 children who did not receive an MMR vaccine.

- Children were significantly more likely to develop joint and limb symptoms within 6 weeks following MMR vaccination compared with children who did not receive MMR (relative risk, RR = 1.6). Specific joint syndromes were nearly 5 times more likely in MMR-vaccinated children (RR = 4.7).

- Girls were significantly more likely to develop joint and limb symptoms for the first time ever within 6 weeks following MMR vaccination when compared with girls who did not receive MMR (RR = 3.5).

- MMR-vaccinated children under 5 years of age were 12 times more likely to develop joint and limb symptoms for the first time ever when compared with children under 5 who did not receive MMR (RR = 12.0).

- Although joint and limb symptoms after MMR occurred most often in children under age 5 and girls, the most severe cases of arthritis were in older boys.

339.

Rubella vaccine recipients are up to 12 times more likely than controls to develop inflammatory arthritis

"The possibility that autoimmunity during the postpartum period may be immunogenetically or hormonally (or both) regulated has implications for rubella immunization strategies in female adults."

Mitchell LA, Tingle AJ, et al. **HLA-DR class II associations with rubella vaccine-induced joint manifestations.** *J Infect Dis* 1998 Jan; 177(1): 5-12.

• Study results show that rubella vaccine recipients are nearly twice as likely as placebo recipients to develop arthropathy (odds ratio, OR = 1.9).

• Results also indicate that certain DR2 and DR5 alleles (genetic mutations) may increase susceptibility to joint disorders such as arthralgia and arthritis following rubella vaccination.

340.

Pattison E, Harrison BJ, et al. **Environmental risk factors for the development of psoriatic arthritis: results from a case-control study.** *Ann Rheum Dis* 2008 May; 67(5): 672-76.

• This study compared 98 patients with psoriasis and inflammatory arthritis to 163 patients with psoriasis but no arthritis.

• Patients with inflammatory arthritis were 12 times more likely than controls to have been vaccinated against rubella prior to onset of the debilitating ailment (odds ratio, OR = 12.4).

341.

The rubella vaccine significantly elevates the risk of acute and chronic arthritis

"The development of arthralgia or arthritis or both in 27% of adult females receiving RA 27/3 rubella vaccine is consistent with results obtained in previously published reports. The onset of joint symptoms at a mean of 17 days post-immunization and the principal involvement of knee, wrist, ankle, and the metacarpophalangeal joints is also typical of the post-vaccine, rubella-associated arthritis syndrome."

Tingle AJ, Yang T, et al. **Prospective immunological assessment of arthritis induced by rubella vaccine.** *Infect Immun* 1983 Apr; 40(1): 22-28.

- In this study, 11% of adult females who received a rubella vaccine (RA 27/3 strain) developed arthritis with multiple recurrent episodes of joint effusion or swelling that lasted at least 6 months (the length of the follow-up period). Another 16% of vaccinated women developed transient arthralgia.

- The presence of rubella antibodies pre-vaccine may enhance the development and/or severity of arthritis post-vaccine.

342.

Tingle AJ, Mitchell LA, et al. **Randomised double-blind placebo-controlled study on adverse effects of rubella immunisation in sero-negative women.** *Lancet* 1997 May 3; 349(9061): 1277-81.

- In this randomized double-blind, placebo-controlled study, 546 women were divided into two groups and received a rubella vaccine (RA27/3 strain) or saline placebo. Vaccine recipients were significantly more likely than controls to develop acute (OR = 1.73) and chronic (OR = 1.58) arthralgia or arthritis.

343.

Rubella vaccination given around the time of menstruation increases the risk of developing arthritis

"Arthropathy occurred significantly more often in women vaccinated at the progestational stage than in women vaccinated at the estrogenic stage."

Nakazono N, Fujimoto S, et al. **Factors associated with clinical reactions to rubella vaccination in women.** *Int J Gynaecol Obstet* 1987 Jun; 25(3): 207-16.

- In this study, 272 healthy women received a rubella vaccine. They were then tested for clinical reactions associated with antibody response, human leukocyte antigen (HLA) type, basal body temperature, menstrual cycles, and serum progesterone levels.

- Women vaccinated during the phase of the menstrual cycle preceding menstruation (the progestational stage) were significantly more likely to develop arthropathy than women vaccinated during the phase preceding ovulation (the estrogenic stage).

344.

Monto AS, Cavallaro JJ, Whale EH. **Frequency of arthralgia in women receiving one of three rubella vaccines.** *Arch Intern Med* 1970 Oct; 126(4): 635-39.

- Women who receive a rubella vaccine within 5 days before or after the onset of menstruation are five times more likely to develop arthritis than women vaccinated 6 to 24 days after the onset of the last menstrual cycle.

345.

Chronic and recurrent arthritis with neurological sequelae, due to rubella vaccination, is well documented in the medical literature

"Immune responses to rubella virus studied at sequential intervals after vaccination correlated with development of rheumatologic and neurological manifestations."

Tingle AJ, Chantler JK, et al. **Postpartum rubella immunization: association with development of prolonged arthritis, neurological sequelae, and chronic rubella viremia.** *J Infect Dis* 1985 Sep; 152(3): 606-12.

- Six women developed polyarticular arthritis (affecting many joints) within 12 days to three weeks after rubella vaccination and have had chronic or recurrent arthralgia or arthritis for two to seven years after vaccination.

- Three of the women also developed acute neurological manifestations consisting of carpal tunnel syndrome or multiple paresthesia. Two of the women developed chronic recurrent episodes of blurred vision and paresthesia after rubella vaccination.

346.

Mitchell LA, Tingle AJ, et al. **Chronic rubella vaccine-associated arthropathy.** *Arch Intern Med* 1993 Oct 11; 153(19): 2268-74.

"Rubella immunization or infection should be considered as additional causative factors in evaluation of acute and continuing musculoskeletal syndromes."

- After rubella vaccination, two women developed polyarthralgia, arthritis, maculopapular rash, fever, paresthesia, and malaise with persistent or recurrent manifestations lasting more than two years.

347.

Hepatitis B vaccination sextuples the risk of arthritis in children

"Evidence from this study suggests that hepatitis B vaccine is positively associated with adverse health outcomes in the general population of U.S. children."

Fisher MA, Eklund SA, et al. **Adverse events associated with hepatitis B vaccine in U.S. children less than six years of age, 1993 and 1994.** *Ann Epidemiol* 2001 Jan; 11(1): 13-21.

• This study evaluated adverse reactions to the hepatitis B vaccine in 12,020 children less than 6 years of age by analyzing datasets from the National Health Interview Survey (health data collected by the U.S. Census Bureau).

• Controlling for age, race, and gender, the hepatitis B vaccine was found to be significantly associated with arthritis in children (odds ratio, OR = 5.91).

348.

Maillefert JF, Sibilia J, et al. **Rheumatic disorders developed after hepatitis B vaccination.** *Rheumatology (Oxford)* 1999 Oct;38(10):978-83.

• Researchers documented 22 people who developed rheumatic disorders within two months following hepatitis B vaccination. Diagnoses included rheumatoid arthritis, post-vaccinal arthritis, and polyarthralgia/myalgia.

• None of the patients had a previously diagnosed rheumatic disease.

349.

Gross K, Combe C, et al. **Arthritis after hepatitis B vaccination. Report of three cases.** *Scand J Rheumatol* 1995; 24(1): 50-52.

"These three cases show that arthritis after hepatitis B vaccination probably is more common than reported so far, especially in a genetically predisposed subject."

350.

The Covid vaccine increases the risk of arthritis and other joint-related adverse effects

"Patients with COVID-19 vaccination-related new-onset arthritis, arthralgias, joint disease flare-up, and bursitis usually present with swelling, pain, stiffness, and, occasionally, decreased range of motion of the affected joint."

> Dawoud R, Haddad D, et al. **COVID-19 vaccine-related arthritis: a descriptive study of case reports on a rare complication.** *Cureus* 2022 Jul 9; 14(7): e26702.

- This paper reviewed 16 case reports of joint-related adverse effects that occurred shortly after covid-19 vaccination.

- Joint-related adverse effects following covid-19 vaccination include septic arthritis, rheumatoid arthritis, acute reactive arthritis, Still's disease, poly-arthritis of the hand, ankle, knee, elbow and shoulder joints, and bursitis.

- In some cases, onset of joint-related adverse events occurred as early as within 30 minutes, 12 hours, 2 days, 3 days, or 1 week after covid vaccination. All cases occurred within 3 weeks post-vaccination.

- Joint-related adverse effects occurred after the following covid vaccines: Pfizer, AstraZeneca, Moderna, Sinovac, Sputnik, and Covaxin.

- Two markers of inflammation—erythrocyte sedimentation rate (ESR) and C-reactive protein (CRP)—were elevated.

- The authors hypothesize that vaccines containing inactivated or attenuated viral pathogens may trigger autoimmune disease. With mRNA vaccines (Pfizer and Moderna), a similar process may occur triggered by viral antigens produced by host cells. Adjuvants could also provoke autoimmune reactions.

- Healthcare workers should be attentive to patients with joint pain, swelling, and stiffness that occurs within a week subsequent to covid vaccination.

351.

Covid vaccination increases the risk of arthritis

"In this systematic review, we studied newly induced arthritis following COVID-19 vaccination."

Liu J, Wu H, Xia S. **New-onset arthritis following COVID-19 vaccination: a systematic review of case reports.** *Vaccines (Basel)* 2023 Mar 15; 11(3): 665.

- This study investigated 45 cases of new-onset arthritis after covid vaccination. Patients were 17 to 90 years of age; 67% were women.

- Of all patients, 64% developed symptoms after the first dose, 67% within the first week post-vaccination, and 71% developed arthritis in multiple joints.

- Diagnoses included rheumatoid arthritis, reactive arthritis, septic arthritis, inflammatory arthritis, and adult-onset Still's disease. Symptoms included joint swelling, joint pain, and limited range of motion.

352.

Golstein MA, Fagnart O, Steinfeld SD. **Reactive arthritis after COVID-19 vaccination: 17 cases.** *Rheumatology (Oxford)* 2023 Nov 2; 62(11): 3706-09.

"The ankle bi-arthritis occurrence chronology, the follow-up and the similar clinical presentation might suggest a pathogenic role of RNA vaccination."

- The authors of this paper documented 17 cases of ankle arthritis that occurred shortly after mRNA covid vaccination.

- Of the 17 patients, 13 (82%) were in women. The arthritis occurred on average 10 days after the first dose and 16 days after the second dose.

- All patients tested positive for covid spike antibodies, suggesting that over-reactive immunity to the vaccine spike protein may have triggered the arthritis.

353.

After covid vaccination, new cases and reactivations of arthritis and psoriasis are possible

"The present result suggests that for some rheumatoid arthritis patients, the SARS-CoV-2 vaccine might act as a potential trigger for exacerbation of arthritis compared with healthy individuals."

Takatani A, Iwamoto N, et al. **Impact of SARS-CoV-2 mRNA vaccine on arthritis condition in rheumatoid arthritis.** *Front Immunol* 2023 Aug 15; 14: 1256655.

• The authors compared the frequency and duration of post-covid vaccination arthralgia (joint pain) between 1198 rheumatoid arthritis patients and controls. Compared with controls, rheumatoid arthritis patients developed joint pain more frequently, it was longer lasting, and they required more drugs.

354.

Wojturska W, Nowakowski J, et al. **Reactive arthritis after vaccination against SARS-CoV-2: a case series and a mini-review.** *Hum Vaccin Immunother* 2023 Dec 31; 19(1): 2173912.

• Besides arthritis, other autoimmune and rheumatic diseases after covid vaccination have been widely described in the literature.

355.

Wu P, Huang I, et al. **New onset and exacerbations of psoriasis following COVID-19 vaccines: a systematic review.** *Am J Clin Dermatol* 2022 Nov; 23(6): 775-799.

"Both new-onset psoriasis and psoriasis flares were reported as cutaneous adverse events following COVID-19 vaccination."

• The authors reviewed 11 studies with 314 cases of new-onset psoriasis or flares after covid vaccination. Psoriasis occurred 1 to 90 days post-vaccination.

The Microbiome

The microbiome is the community of microorganisms, such as fungi, bacteria and viruses, that live on our bodies and inside us. These groups of microorganisms are mutable and change in response to environmental factors, such as diet, medication, and exercise. Your microbiome includes both "good" and "bad" microbes. Although the microbes are very small and can only be seen by a microscope, they contribute in important ways to human health and wellness.

The studies in this chapter discuss how the microbiome can benefit health and increase vaccine efficacy. Children born in undernourished settings with poor sanitation and greater intestinal disease burden have deficient immune responses to vaccination when compared to children in developed nations. Probiotics improve vaccine efficacy by stimulating the immune system and can facilitate a return to homeostasis following a disease challenge.

The type, diversity, quantity, and quality of gut microbiota are contributors to the variable efficacy of vaccines. But vaccine efficacy is only one factor affected by the composition of your microbiome. According to both Ng and Yuan, an unhealthy, imbalanced microbiome might also contribute to vaccine adverse reactions. Ng also found that low immunity after covid vaccination was correlated with an abundance of *B. vulgatus* and *B. thetaiotaomicron* prior to vaccination. And among covid vaccine recipients, those with any adverse event after the first dose had a significant decrease in bacterial species richness.

356.

Optimal composition of the intestinal ecosystem benefits health and increases vaccine efficacy

"The ever-expanding information on how the microbiota shapes the immune system will have a profound impact on the future of vaccines, requiring a major shift in our current approach to vaccine development."

Valdez Y, Brown EM, Finlay BB. **Influence of the microbiota on vaccine effectiveness.** *Trends Immunol* 2014 Nov; 35(11): 526-37.

- Humans have co-evolved for millions of years with our microbiota in a symbiotic relationship that is essential for health. This paper summarizes recent literature on the composition of the intestinal ecosystem and its influence on vaccine immune responses.

- Three major environmental factors affect microbiota in early life: birth method (vaginal vs. Caesarean), diet (breastfed vs. formula-fed), and hygiene (clean vs. unsanitary). These differences in early-life microbiota composition will influence the child's immune response to vaccines.

- Children born in undernourished settings with poor sanitation and greater intestinal disease burden have deficient immune responses to vaccination when compared to children in developed nations.

- Nutrition influences the adaptive immune system. Many micronutrients are essential for healthy immune function and vaccine effectiveness. Malnutrition alters the microbiome and may "predispose a host to intestinal damage and immune defects that are negatively correlated to vaccine outcome."

- Probiotics may improve vaccine efficacy by stimulating the immune system and can facilitate a return to homeostasis following a disease challenge.

- Antibiotics disrupt microbial diversity. A more diverse intestinal microbiota may provide a better immune response to certain vaccines, indicating a need for scientists to consider microbiota composition during human vaccine trials.

357.

The status of intestinal microbes may influence vaccine efficacy

"A major implication of our findings for global public health is the possibility that the microbiota plays a role in immune responses to vaccines. The status of the host microbiota may be a critical determinant of vaccine efficacy."

Oh JZ, Ravindran R, et al. **TLR5-mediated sensing of gut microbiota is necessary for antibody responses to seasonal influenza vaccination.** *Immunity* 2014 Sep 18; 41(3): 478-492.

- It is unclear why a significant proportion of vaccinated people remain susceptible to infection and why vaccines are less effective in developing countries. This paper examined the possibility that the intestinal microbiota influences antibody responses to vaccination.

- Scientists compared vaccine-induced immune responses between germ-free mice (devoid of microbes) and specific-pathogen free mice (free of germs that can cause disease). The germ-free mice had significantly reduced immune responses. Re-establishment of the microbiota promotes antibody responses.

- Healthy mice were given antibiotics until 95% of fecal bacteria were eliminated. The mice were then vaccinated. Vaccine immunity following depletion of the intestinal microbiota was substantially reduced but steadily increased by 4 weeks post-vaccination to amounts similar in untreated mice.

- The TLR5 gene mediates between flagellin — a specific type of bacteria derived from the microbiota — and the induction of antibodies to inactivated influenza and polio vaccines. (Flagellin appears to act as a natural adjuvant.)

- These studies indicate that the intestinal microbiota is crucial for the rapid induction of antibody responses following vaccination.

- The findings in this paper suggest that diet, nutrition, metabolic diseases, gut-associated pathologies, and other factors affecting the microbiota may significantly influence antibody responses to current and future vaccines.

358.

The type, diversity, quantity, and quality of gut microbiota are contributors to the variable efficacy of vaccines

"Understanding how different compositions of microbiota interact with various immune cells could open new insights into vaccine design."

Lex JR, Azizi A. **Microbiota, a forgotten relic of vaccination.** *Expert Rev Vaccines* 2017 Dec; 16(12): 1171-73.

• Vaccines have variable efficacy, most notably in developing versus developed countries. This paper reviewed factors that influence composition of the human gut microbiota and their impact on vaccine immune responses.

• Proper gut microbiota composition is protective against infections and also is crucial in inducing an adequate immune response following vaccination.

• Probiotics bolster the gut microbiota while antibiotics disrupt microbial diversity, requiring weeks or months for a return to normal.

359.

Harris VC, Armah G, et al. **Significant correlation between the infant gut microbiome and rotavirus vaccine response in rural Ghana.** *J Infect Dis* 2017 Jan1; 215(1): 34-41.

"The intestinal microbiome composition correlates significantly with rotavirus vaccine immunogenicity and may contribute to the diminished vaccine immunogenicity observed in developing countries."

• This study analyzed pre-vaccination fecal microbiome compositions in 78 infants in rural Ghana who had either sufficient or poor immune responses to rotavirus vaccination (responders and non-responders). Their microbiomes were then compared with the microbiomes of 154 healthy Dutch infants.

• Ghana responders had microbiomes that were significantly more similar to the microbiomes of Dutch infants than to Ghana non-responders.

360.

Vaccine-induced immune responses are influenced by the intestinal microbiome

"Given the growing list of ways that the microbiome can influence the immune system, it would be surprising if the microbiome did not also influence vaccine responses."

Lynn DJ, Pulendran B. **The potential of the microbiota to influence vaccine responses.** *J Leukoc Biol* 2018 Feb; 103(2): 225-31.

• Humans are inhabited by an extensive group of microorganisms. The intestinal microbiome contains a great diversity of microbes that perform essential functions, including the metabolism of nutrients, the maintenance of gut homeostasis, and the regulation of gut mucosal immunity.

• This paper summarized the scientific evidence that the intestinal microbiome is a significant factor influencing immune responses to vaccination.

361.

Williams WB, Han Q, Haynes BF. **Cross-reactivity of HIV vaccine responses and the microbiome.** *Curr Opin HIV AIDS* 2018 Jan; 13(1): 9-14.

• This paper found that the microbiome can divert HIV-vaccine-induced antibody responses away from protective immunity, just one of several obstacles to creating an effective vaccine against HIV.

362.

Tarabichi Y, Li K, et al. **The administration of intranasal live attenuated influenza vaccine induces changes in the nasal microbiota and nasal epithelium gene expression profiles.** *Microbiome* 2015 Dec 15; 3: 74.

"We found that live attenuated influenza vaccination led to significant changes in microbial community structure, diversity, and core taxonomic membership as well as increases in the relative abundances of Staphylococcus and Bacteroides genera."

363.

Composition of the microbiome influences health and vaccine immune responses

"It is well established that gut microbiota can affect mucosal immune function...but the present observation of an equally strong association of stool microbiota with response to parenteral vaccination is, we believe, novel."

Huda MN, Lewis Z, et al. **Stool microbiota and vaccine responses of infants.** *Pediatrics* 2014 Aug; 134(2): e362-72.

• Vaccine efficacy is low in less-developed nations, possibly due to intestinal dysbiosis, a condition in which gut bacteria are out of balance. This study was conducted to determine if the composition of stool microbiota could predict vaccine immune responses.

• Scientists analyzed the stool microbiota of 48 Bangladeshi infants. One particular strain of bacteria predominated and was positively associated with T-cell responses to the oral polio, tuberculosis, and tetanus vaccines, while three other strains were associated with lower vaccine responses.

• Right composition of the gut microbiota promotes infant health and optimal development of the immune system. Vaccine immune responsiveness may be advanced by minimizing dysbiosis early in infancy.

364.

Salk HM, Simon WL, et al. **Taxa of the nasal microbiome are associated with influenza-specific IgA response to live attenuated influenza vaccine.** *PloS One* 2016 Sep 19; 11(9): e0162803.

• The live attenuated influenza vaccination induced alterations to the nasal microbiome. Some changes were associated with a significant increase in H1-specific antibody titers while other changes correlated with significantly decreased H3-specific immune responses.

365.

Probiotic bacteria have immune-stimulating properties that increase vaccine efficacy

"Probiotics may be a novel strategy to enhance the protection afforded by current vaccines, particularly in developing countries where the disease risk is greatest."

Licciardi PV, Tang ML. **Vaccine adjuvant properties of probiotic bacteria.** *Discov Med* 2011 Dec; 12(67): 525-33.

- Probiotics are live microorganisms that when administered or consumed confer health benefits to the host. Their combined effect on gut microbiota and immune modulation — interactions between the microbiota and immune system — are important for the development of healthy immune responses.

- This paper reviewed evidence supporting the use of probiotic bacteria as novel mucosal adjuvants to enhance existing vaccine-specific immune responses.

366.

Davidson LE, Fiorino A, et al. **Lactobacillus GG as an immune adjuvant for live attenuated influenza vaccine in healthy adults: a randomized double blind placebo controlled trial.** *Eur J Clin Nutr* 2011 April; 65(4): 501-507.

"Lactobacillus GG has potential as an important adjuvant to improve influenza vaccine immunogenicity."

- In a randomized, double-blind, placebo-controlled study 39 healthy adults received a live influenza vaccine. They were then randomized to either receive a probiotic or placebo twice daily for 4 weeks. Antibody titers were measured prior to vaccination (baseline), on day 28 and day 56.

- Antibody titers for the H3N2 influenza strain were significantly higher in the probiotic group compared to the placebo group on day 28. They also were higher on day 56 although not statistically significant.

367.

Consumption of probiotic bacteria improves vaccine efficacy

"Probiotics induce an immunologic response that may provide enhanced systemic protection of cells from virus infections by increasing production of virus neutralizing antibodies."

de Vrese M, Rautenberg P, et al. **Probiotic bacteria stimulate virus-specific neutralizing antibodies following a booster polio vaccination.** *Eur J Nutr* 2005 Oct; 44(7): 406-13.

- In a randomized, double-blind, placebo-controlled study 64 people consumed for 5 weeks clotted milk with or without probiotic bacteria (the treatment and control groups). In the second week, everyone received an oral polio vaccine. Immune responses were measured before and after vaccination.

- The group that received probiotics had poliovirus neutralizing antibody titers that were 2 to 4-fold higher than the group that received a placebo.

368.

Rizzardini G, Eskesen D, et al. **Evaluation of the immune benefits of two probiotic strains...in an influenza vaccination model: a randomised, double-blind, placebo-controlled study.** *Br J Nutr* 2012 Mar;107(6): 876-84.

"Data herein show that supplementation with [probiotic strain 1 or strain 2] may be an effective means to improve immune function by augmenting systemic and mucosal immune responses to challenge."

- In a randomized, double-blind, placebo-controlled study 211 people consumed for 6 weeks a probiotic capsule (strain 1) or probiotic dairy drink (strain 2) or placebo. After the second week, everyone received an influenza vaccine. Immune responses were measured before and after vaccination.

- Antibody titers were significantly greater than baseline in both groups that received a probiotic compared to the placebo group.

369.

Probiotic supplementation significantly enhances vaccine immune responses

"Oral administration of [probiotic bacteria] potentates the immuno-logic response of an anti-influenza vaccine and may provide enhanced systemic protection from infection by increasing the T-helper type 1 response and virus-neutralizing antibodies."

Olivares M, Díaz-Ropero MP, et al. **Oral intake of *Lactobacillus fermentum* CECT5716 enhances the effects of influenza vaccination.** *Nutrition* 2007 Mar; 23(3): 254-60.

- In a randomized, placebo-controlled study 50 people received probiotic bacteria or placebo for 4 weeks. Two weeks later, they received an influenza vaccine. Two weeks after vaccination, immune responses were measured.

- Immune responses were significantly higher in the group that received probiotic supplementation. This group also had a lower incidence of influenza-like illness during the 5 months after vaccination.

370.

Maidens C, Childs C, et al. **Modulation of vaccine response by concomitant probiotic administration.** *Br J Clin Pharmacol* 2013 Mar; 75(3): 663-70.

"Evidence that gut-resident bacteria play a role in shaping immune defenses form the basis for the hypothesis that probiotics may modulate responses to infection or vaccination."

371.

Soh SE, Ong DQ, et al. **Effect of probiotic supplementation in the first 6 months of life on specific antibody responses to infant hepatitis B vaccination.** *Vaccine* 2010 Mar 19; 28(14): 2577-79.

"Probiotics may enhance specific antibody responses in infants receiving certain hepatitis B vaccine schedules."

372.

Probiotics significantly enhance vaccine immune responses in the elderly

"These studies demonstrate that daily consumption of this particular probiotic product increased relevant specific antibody responses to influenza vaccination in individuals of over 70 years of age and may therefore provide a health benefit in this population."

Boge T, Rémigy M, et al. **A probiotic fermented dairy drink improves antibody response to influenza vaccination in the elderly in two randomised controlled trials.** *Vaccine* 2009 Sep 18; 27(41): 5677-84.

- In two randomized, double-blind, controlled studies 86 and 222 healthy seniors over 70 years of age consumed a probiotic dairy drink or placebo twice daily for 7 weeks or 13 weeks. Four weeks after starting the regimen, they received an influenza vaccine. Antibody titers were measured post-vaccination.

- In the first study, immune responses were higher in the probiotic group. In the larger study, antibody titers against the B strain of influenza increased significantly more in the probiotic group at 3, 6, and 9 weeks, and 5 months post-vaccine. Results were similar for the H3N2 and H1N1 influenza strains.

373.

Bunout D, Barrera G, et al. **Effects of a nutritional supplement on the immune response and cytokine production in free-living Chilean elderly.** *J Parenter Enteral Nutr* 2004 Sep-Oct; 28(5): 348-54.

"This nutritional supplement increased innate immunity and protection against infections in elderly people."

- Sixty healthy seniors at least 70 years of age were studied. Half received a daily nutritional supplement that included probiotic bacteria. After 4 months, everyone received influenza and pneumococcal vaccines. Immune responses were measured at various intervals post-vaccination.

- Immune responses were higher in supplemented subjects compared to the controls. Supplemented subjects also reported significantly fewer infections.

374.

Probiotic bacteria protect mice against influenza

"These results demonstrate that oral administration of selected lactobacilli might protect host animals from flu infection by interactions with gut immunity."

Kawase M, He F, et al. **Oral administration of lactobacilli from human intestinal tract protects mice against influenza virus infection.** *Lett Appl Microbiol* 2010 Jul; 51(1): 6-10.

- In this study, 39 mice were orally administered either probiotic bacteria or placebo for 19 days. On day 14, they were infected with the influenza virus, and their clinical symptoms were monitored. After 6 days of infection, the mice were killed and pulmonary virus titers were measured.

- The "clinical symptom" scores of the probiotic-fed mice were significantly better compared to those of the control mice, and pulmonary virus titers of the probiotic-fed mice were significantly decreased.

375.

Harata G, He F, et al. **Intranasal administration of** *Lactobacillus rhamnosus* **GG protects mice from H1N1 influenza virus infection by regulating respiratory immune responses.** *Lett Appl Microbiol* 2010 Jun 1; 50(6): 597-602.

"We have demonstrated that probiotics might protect host animals from viral infection by stimulating immune responses in the respiratory tract."

- In this study, 26 mice were infected with the influenza virus after half of them were intranasally exposed to probiotic bacteria for 3 days. Morbidity and mortality of the infected mice were monitored for 2 weeks.

- Mice treated with probiotic bacteria had a significantly lower accumulated symptom rate and a significantly higher survival rate than control mice.

376.

Recent use of antibiotics is associated with reduced covid vaccine efficacy

"Our current study is the first to report an association between the usage of antibiotics and impaired early vaccine immunogenicity after one dose of BNT162b2 [Pfizer covid vaccine]. Our results shed light on the potential interaction between gut microbiota and vaccine immunogenicity."

> Cheung K, Lam L, et al. **Association between recent usage of antibiotics and immunogenicity within six months after COVID-19 vaccination.** *Vaccines* (Basel) 2022 Jul 14; 10(7): 1122.

- This study investigated whether antibiotic use within the prior six months influences covid vaccine immunogenicity (i.e., efficacy).

- Covid vaccine recipients who used antibiotics during the prior six months were compared to covid vaccine recipients who were non-antibiotic users. Antibiotic users had lower seroconversion rates (i.e., reduced immune protection) at 3 weeks ($p = 0.14$) and 8 weeks ($p = 0.15$) post-vaccination.

- A multivariate analysis revealed that recent antibiotic usage was associated with a statistically significantly 74% lower immune response at 3 weeks post-vaccination (adjusted odds ratio, aOR = 0.26, CI: 0.08-0.96). Male sex and older age were also associated with significantly lower immune responses.

- Since antibiotics are known to cause gut dysbiosis, and the composition and function of gastrointestinal microbiota are now recognized as important factors that modulate immune responses to several vaccines, it's not surprising that antibiotic use may reduce covid-19 vaccine efficacy.

- Antibiotic-induced disturbance of gut microbiota may take several months to recover. This might explain why immune responses in antibiotic users at 6 months post-vaccination were not lower than non-antibiotic users.

- Vaccinated antibiotic users also had a higher rate of "systemic adverse reaction of vomiting" when compared to antibiotic non-users ($p = 0.04$).

377.

Antibiotic use in young children is associated with reduced immune responses to several childhood vaccines

"Antibiotic use in children less than 2 years of age is associated with lower vaccine-induced antibody levels to several vaccines."

Chapman TJ, Pham M, et al. **Antibiotic use and vaccine antibody levels.** *Pediatrics* 2022 May 1; 149(5): e2021052061.

- Most children are prescribed antibiotics in the first year of life, but data are scarce regarding its affect on vaccine-induced immunity.

- In this study of 560 children 6 to 24 months of age, researchers measured antibody levels after several vaccines were administered to 342 children with, and 218 without, antibiotic prescriptions.

- At 9-24 months of age, children who had received antibiotics were significantly more likely than children who had received no antibiotics to have non-protective vaccine-induced antibody levels to several pertussis and pneumococcal antigens ($p < .05$).

- At 9-12 months of age, children who took antibiotics had a greater frequency of non-protective antibody levels associated with several vaccines ($p < .05$).

- The number of antibiotic courses in the first year of life had an effect on subsequent vaccine-induced antibody levels. Each antibody course reduced median antibody levels to inactivated polio, pneumococcal, Hib, and DTaP vaccines by 11.3%, 10.4%, 6.8%, and 5.8%, respectively (all $p \leq .05$).

- The effect of accumulated antibiotics was worse after booster shots at 18-24 months of age. Each antibody prescription reduced antibody levels by 21.3% for Hib, 18.9% for polio, 18.1% for DTaP, and 12.2% for pneumococcus.

- Prior research indicates that antibiotics alter the composition of bacteria in the gut microbiome which can impact vaccine immune responses.

378.

Type of birth (vaginal vs. cesarean) affects early life gut microbiota composition and vaccine immune responses

"We demonstrate that mode of delivery-induced differences in the gut microbiota in the first weeks of life [vaginal delivery versus cesarean], including differences in E. coli and Bifidobacterium relative abundances, are associated with anti-pneumococcal and anti-meningitis C IgG [antibody] responses to vaccination."

de Koff EM, van Baarle D, et al. **Mode of delivery modulates the intestinal microbiota and impacts the response to vaccination.** *Nat Commun* 2022 Nov 15; 13(1): 6638.

- Previous studies have shown that immune responses to some vaccines (e.g., hepatitis B, tetanus, BCG, oral polio, and oral rotavirus) may be influenced by the composition of the microbial environment prior to vaccination.

- In this study of 120 healthy, term born infants, the authors investigated associations between early life exposures, gut microbiota composition in early life, and vaccine immune responses several months later.

- Vaginal birth was associated with a relative abundance of beneficial bacteria in early life. High abundances of *Bifidobacterium* and *E. coli* during the first weeks after birth were associated with robust antibody responses to pneumo-coccal and meningococcal vaccines at 12 and 18 months of life, respectively.

- Immune responses to pneumococcal and meningococcal vaccines are more robust in vaginal versus cesarean births.

- The positive effect of a vaginal birth was diminished by formula feeding. For example, pneumococcal vaccine antibody levels in the vaginally-delivered infants were 3.5 times higher in breastfed vs. formula-fed infants.

- Vaccine antibody responses were more greatly correlated to microbiota composition in early life rather than closer to the time of vaccination.

379.

Microbiome composition is associated with covid vaccine immunity and adverse events

"We found that baseline gut microbiota was significantly associated with immunogenicity and adverse events of COVID-19 vaccines."

Ng SC, Peng Y, et al. **Gut microbiota composition is associated with SARS-CoV-2 vaccine immunogenicity and adverse events.** *Gut* 2022 Jun; 71(6): 1106-1116.

- This study examined gut microbiota composition in 138 adults before and after they received two doses of either an inactivated or mRNA covid vaccine for associations with vaccine-related immune responses and adverse events.

- Baseline gut microbiome composition predicts immune response one month post-vaccination. For example, low immunity post-vaccine was correlated with an abundance of *B. vulgatus* and *B. thetaiotaomicron* pre-vaccine.

- Gut microbiome composition is associated with vaccine-related adverse events. Among mRNA covid vaccine recipients, those with any adverse event after the first dose had a significant decrease in bacterial species richness.

- The beneficial effect of four bacterial species, and immune responses, were compromised in overweight and obese people.

380.

Yuan L, Tsai P, Bell K. **Do gut microbiota mediate adverse vaccine reaction?** *Ann Clin Trials Vaccines Res* 2018; 2(2): 11-12.

"Studies may demonstrate how an 'unhealthy,' imbalanced microbiome contributes to an adverse vaccine reaction, and also how 'healthy' microbiota may be protective against injury."

- The authors of this paper propose a study with the central hypothesis that an absence of protective gut microbiota coupled with an overgrowth of pathogenic strains significantly affect host response to vaccination, establishing a microbial predisposition to an adverse vaccine reaction.

Birth Control

An estimated 80 million women have unintended pregnancies worldwide annually, so scientists would like to develop a better method of contraception. Developing contraceptive vaccines is challenging because they must be safe, long-lasting, and reversible. Also, they will be used by healthy people and require close to 100% efficacy.

Contraceptive vaccines that produce anti-sperm antibodies are in development. Researchers have also created a birth control vaccine that induces an immune attack against human chorionic gonadotropin (hCG), a pregnancy hormone. In phase 2 clinical trials, sexually active women were given 3 injections of an anti-hCG vaccine at 6-week intervals. Eighty percent of these women developed antibody titers at levels considered protective against pregnancy.

The World Health Organization (WHO) has been researching and developing birth control vaccines since 1972, when it initiated studies on ways to prevent an embryo from adhering to the uterus. Shortly thereafter, WHO established the *Task Force on Immunological Methods for the Regulation of Fertility* to find ways to prevent implantation, inhibit sperm transport and fertilization, and hinder blastocyst hatching through interference with the zona pellucida.

There is opposition to research on birth control vaccines. Some people believe that when anti-fertility vaccines become more widely available, nations may be tempted to regulate fertility. Scientists who develop birth control vaccines stress their advantages while women who might use them cite disadvantages, including side-effects and the potential for misuse by population control programs.

Some researchers claim that fertile women in several developing nations might have already received an anti-fertility vaccine without their consent. For example, a recent paper provides evidence that from 2013-2015, pregnant females in Kenya received multiple doses of a vaccine that they believed would protect their babies against neonatal tetanus. However, the dosage schedule was most appropriate for an anti-fertility vaccine but inappropriate for a tetanus toxoid vaccine.

There are valid concerns about the safety and ethics of giving women immune-stimulating birth control vaccines. If an immune response to the reproductive antigen persists, it could result in ovarian dysfunction and permanent infertility. Scientists also seek to prevent anti-fertility vaccines from causing autoimmune disease, and are monitoring for birth defects (when the mother halts contraception and becomes pregnant). Anti-fertility vaccines involve both the reproductive and immune systems so it is imperative that they are proven safe over an extended period of time prior to being licensed for use in fertile populations.

381.

Contraceptive vaccines that produce anti-sperm antibodies are in development

"Recent advances in the fields of vaccinology, adjuvants, and nano-technology will help to expedite contraceptive vaccine development."

Naz RK. **Vaccine for human contraception targeting sperm Izumo protein and YLP12 dodecamer peptide.** *Protein Sci* 2014 Jul; 23(7): 857-68.

- An estimated 80 million women have unintended pregnancies worldwide annually, so scientists would like to develop a better method of contraception.

- Developing contraceptive vaccines is challenging because they must be safe, long-lasting, and reversible. Also, they will be used by healthy people and require close to 100% efficacy.

- Animal and human studies have shown that immunizing males and females with sperm produces anti-sperm antibodies that result in contraception. However, whole sperm cannot be used; only sperm-specific proteins can be used to develop sperm-targeted contraceptive vaccines.

- More than 100 sperm-specific proteins have been identified. This paper reviews the development of contraceptive vaccines using two sperm-specific proteins: Izumo protein and YLP_{12} dodecamer peptide.

- In studies of female mice, vaccination with Izumo peptides that were conjugated to various carrier proteins induced reversible contraception.

- In another study, female mice received a vaccine prepared by conjugating synthetic YLP_{12} peptide with recombinant cholera toxin as a carrier protein and adjuvant. The mice had a significant reduction in litter size.

- DNA anti-fertility vaccines may be feasible alternatives to peptide vaccines. They tend to enhance Th1 immune response resulting in secretion of cytokines that negatively affect gamete and embryo function.

- Development of a contraceptive vaccine for human use is a top priority of the World Health Organization.

382.

Scientists are creating sperm-immobilizing antibodies to passively immunize women against pregnancy

"Exploitation of sperm antigens as an immunocontraceptive agent... can result in potent immunocontraception."

Kaur K, Prabha V. **Immunocontraceptives: new approaches to fertility control.** *Biomed Re Int* 2014; 2014: 868196.

- Immuno-contraception is a passive immunization birth control method that aims to block male and female gametes (sperm and egg) from fusing. This paper reviewed the current research on immuno-contraceptive vaccines that utilize sperm-immobilizing antibodies to prevent fertilization.

- The idea of using passive immunization for immuno-contraception originated from clinical reports of infertile men whose semen contained antibodies that immobilize sperm. Sperm-immobilizing antibodies must be present in the vagina to provide a significant immuno-protective effect against pregnancy.

- Passive immunization occurs when an individual receives a preparation containing high concentrations of antibodies against a particular pathogen or other target, such as sperm-specific antigens. For example, vaginal gels may be used for the delivery of sustained-release, anti-sperm antibodies.

- Scientists have isolated several sperm-specific antigens that could be targeted for the development of antibodies that prevent fertilization, including Fertilization Antigen-1 (FA-1), Epididymal Protease Inhibitor (Eppin), A-kinase Anchoring Protein (AHKAP), and Testis Specific Antigen-1 (TSA-1).

- Bacterial pathogens associated with genito-urinary infections, such as *Chlamydia trachomatis, Neisseria gonorrhoeae, E. coli,* and *Staphylococcus aureus,* are known to induce sperm immobilization, and may be exploited for the development of an immuno-contraceptive.

- Novel procedures such as subtractive hybridization and gene knockout technology are being utilized in the search for an ideal immuno-contraceptive.

383.

Scientists isolated a sperm-immobilizing factor from E. coli to create anti-sperm antibodies as a vaginal contraceptive

"Sperm agglutinating factor isolated from E. coli was capable of causing sperm agglutination in vitro and infertility in vivo."

Kaur K, Kaur S, Prabha V. **Exploitation of sperm-*Escherichia coli* interaction at the receptor-ligand level for the development of anti-receptor antibodies as the vaginal contraceptive.** *Andrology* 2015 Mar; 3(2): 385-94.

- Earlier research demonstrated that *Escherichia coli (E. coli),* a common bacterium, rapidly adheres to and agglutinates, or immobilizes, sperm.

- In this study, scientists isolated and purified a sperm-immobilizing factor from *E. coli* that was extracted from semen samples of infertile human males. The goal was to generate anti-sperm receptor antibodies that could be studied in vitro (in a culture dish) and in vivo (in organisms) as a contraceptive.

384.

Reddi PP, Castillo JR, et al. **Production in *Escherichia coli*, purification and immunogenicity of acrosomal protein SP-10, a candidate contraceptive vaccine.** *Gene* 1994 Sep 30; 147(2): 189-95.

"To produce large amounts of pure antigen for ongoing studies of the immunogenicity and anti-fertility effects of SP-10, we used an efficient Escherichia coli expression system."

- The World Health Organization's *Task Force on Vaccines for Fertility Regulation* labeled the human sperm antigen, SP-10, as a primary candidate for the development of a contraceptive vaccine.

- This paper describes the process by which the human sperm antigen, SP-10, was synthesized and purified in *E. Coli,* to produce large quantities for use in creating an effective birth control vaccine.

385.

Scientists created a birth control vaccine by genetically fusing *E. coli,* a common bacterium, with hCG, a hormone produced during pregnancy

"A genetically engineered vaccine consisting of beta hCG linked to B subunit of heat labile enterotoxin of E. coli has been made. It is expressed as DNA as well as protein."

Talwar GP, Nand KN, et al. **Current status of a unique vaccine preventing pregnancy.** *Front Biosci* (Elite Ed) 2017 Jun 1; 9(2): 321-32.

• This paper summarizes the status of a new genetically engineered birth control vaccine that combined *Escherichia coli,* a common bacterium, with human chorionic gonadotropin (hCG), a hormone produced during pregnancy.

• Previous studies conducted in India, Finland, Sweden, Chile and Brazil already confirmed the ability of a vaccine that linked hCG with tetanus toxoid to generate antibodies against hCG, and showed that anti-hCG antibody titers above 50 ng/ml prevented pregnancy of sexually active fertile women.

• This new birth control vaccine has been cleared for clinical trials by the *Review Committee on Genetic Manipulation* in India.

386.

Rock EP, Reich KA, et al. **Immunogenicity of a fusion protein linking the beta subunit carboxyl terminal peptide (CTP) of human chorionic gonadotropin to the B subunit of** *Escherichia coli* **heat-labile enterotoxin (LTB).** *Vaccine* 1996 Nov; 14(16): 1560-68.

• Scientists working on an anti-fertility vaccine have engineered a fusion protein consisting of *Escherichia coli* genetically linked to a peptide of human chorionic gonadotropin (hCG).

• Previous anti-fertility vaccine formulations are expensive to produce and require multiple booster shots to maintain effective antibody titers.

387.

Researchers have developed a birth control vaccine that induces an immune attack against the hCG pregnancy hormone

"Immuno-contraception instructs the body to recognize a self-molecule as foreign, so that the body attacks the molecule, thereby affecting contraception."

Koshy LM. **Immuno-contraception undergoing promising trials.** *Indian Med Trib* 1994 Aug 15; 2(13): 7.

• Researchers developing a birth control vaccine have three requirements: the fertility-disrupting target must be crucial for reproduction, the disruption must be transient (so that birth control may be reversed), and antibodies against the target must not cross-react with non-targets in the body.

• Scientists in India have completed phase 2 efficacy trials on a birth control vaccine that successfully linked human chorionic gonadotropin (hCG) with either tetanus or diphtheria toxoid to induce an immune attack against the hCG pregnancy hormone.

• There are two obstacles to overcome: 1) there is a 2-month lapse between the first vaccine dose and the development of sufficient antibody titers to prevent pregnancy, and 2) too many vaccine injections are required.

• A single injection of "biodegradable microcarrier systems" for sustained release of the vaccine might eliminate the need for multiple doses.

388.

Gupta SK, Koothan PT. **Relevance of immuno-contraceptive vaccines for population control. I. hormonal immunocontraception.** *Arch Immunol Ther Exp (Warsz)* 1990; 38(1-2): 47-60.

"Baboons immunized with beta-hCG had shown cross-reactivity to other tissues. Despite these problems and concerns...a decision has been made to proceed with limited clinical trials [on human subjects]."

389.

A birth control vaccine that was developed by genetically linking human and sheep reproductive hormones was tested on 148 fertile women

"This study presents evidence of the feasibility of a vaccine for control of human fertility."

Talwar, GP, Singh O, et al. **A vaccine that prevents pregnancy in women.** *Proc Natl Acad Sci USA* 1994 Aug 30; 91(18): 8532-36.

* Scientists created a birth control vaccine consisting of the hCG pregnancy hormone (human chorionic gonadotropin), conjoined with ovine luteinizing hormone (derived from sheep), conjugated to tetanus and diphtheria toxoids.

* In this phase II clinical trial, 148 sexually active women were given 3 injections of an anti-hCG vaccine at 6-week intervals. Eighty percent of these women developed anti-hCG antibody titers greater than 50ng/ml, a level considered protective against pregnancy.

* The fertile, vaccinated women were observed for a total of 1,224 menstrual cycles; one pregnancy occurred among the 119 women who developed sufficient anti-hCG antibody titers (above 50ng/ml).

390.

Talwar GP, Singh OM, et al. **The HSD-hCG vaccine prevents pregnancy in women: feasibility study of a reversible safe contraceptive vaccine.** *Am J Reprod Immunol* 1997 Feb; 37(2): 153-60.

* Scientists developed a birth control vaccine by genetically conjoining a purified beta subunit of human chorionic gonadotropin (hCG) with a purified alpha subunit of sheep luteinizing hormone (ovine LH) chemically linked to tetanus and diphtheria toxoids. It includes an aluminum adjuvant.

* This paper describes Phase II clinical trials of a reversible birth control vaccine tested on women, and offers strategies for optimizing the vaccine.

391.

A reversible birth control vaccine for women is under development

"This unique vaccine, requiring periodic intake and demonstrating no impairment of ovulation, hormonal profiles and menstrual regularity, is on the verge of final clinical trials under the aegis of the Indian Council of Medical Research and should be a valuable addition to the available contraceptives."

Talwar GP, Gupta JC, et al. **Advances in development of a contraceptive vaccine against human chorionic gonadotropin.** *Expert Opin Biol Ther* 2015; 15(8): 1183-90.

- This paper reviewed historical advancements in the development of a contraceptive vaccine against human chorionic gonadotropin (hCG).

- HCG is a hormone produced during pregnancy. To create a birth control vaccine, scientists sought ways to induce antibodies against hCG.

- To render hCG immunogenic (capable of provoking an immune response), it was conjugated to tetanus toxoid as a carrier. Women who received this vaccine produced antibodies against both hCG and tetanus.

- Further experimentation was required to make the vaccine more immunogenic to obtain higher titers of anti-hCG antibodies without using oily adjuvants.

- In Phase II clinical trials, the vaccine was administered to 148 fertile women who were sexually active. All of the vaccinated women produced anti-hCG antibodies, but only 80% of the women had titers above 50 ng/ml (the protective threshold). One pregnancy occurred in 1224 menstrual cycles.

- Pregnancies occurred when titers dropped below 35 ng/ml, so the vaccinated women received boosters when titers declined below 50 ng/ml.

- A recombinant birth control vaccine linking hCG with *E. coli* was developed. Genetically engineered DNA contraceptive vaccines were tested on marmosets and rodents. Vaccinated animals regained fertility when boosters were halted. Clinical trials on fertile, sexually active women are expected soon.

392.

A birth control vaccine primed with DNA improves its ability to prevent pregnancies

"Immunization with the DNA form of the recombinant hCGβ-LTB vaccine twice at fortnightly interval followed by the proteinic form of the vaccine induces a distinctly higher antibody response."

Nand KN, Gupta JC, et al. **Priming with DNA enhances considerably the immunogenicity of hCG β-LTB vaccine.** *Am J Reprod Immunol* 2015 Oct; 74(4): 302-8.

- This paper provides evidence that priming the recombinant human chorionic gonadotropin (hCG) birth control vaccine with DNA greatly increases the antibody response necessary to prevent women from becoming pregnant.

393.

Wang X, Zhao X, et al. **Gene conjugation of molecular adjuvant C3d3 to hCGbeta increased the anti-hCGbeta Th2 and humoral immune response in DNA immunization.** *J Gene Med* 2006 Apr; 8(4): 498-505.

- DNA immunization is a method to induce an immune response by injecting genetically engineered DNA (that codes for specific proteins) into the body.

- Findings in this study indicate that gene fusion of C3d3 (a protein of the immune system) to hCGbeta (a pregnancy hormone) as a method to stimulate the immune system, may improve the Th2 humoral immune response of the hCGbeta DNA vaccine toward the goal of effective contraception.

394.

Terrazzini N, Hannesdóttir S, et al. **DNA immunization with plasmids expressing hCGbeta-chimeras.** *Vaccine* 2004 Jun 2; 22(17-18): 2146-53.

- This paper discusses the use of DNA immunization to improve the immunogenicity of human chorionic gonadotropin (hCG), a pregnancy hormone used in anti-fertility vaccines.

395.

Birth control vaccines have been under development since the 1970s

"A vaccine capable of causing active immunity against one or more key elements of conception would have several advantages over currently available methods of fertility regulation."

Talwar GP. **The present and future of immunologic approaches to contraception.** *Int J Gynaecol Obstet* 1978; 15(5): 410-14.

• Scientists have begun developing different types of birth control vaccines, including those based on autoimmunity against sperm, anti-zona pellucida, anti-nonhormonal placenta-specific proteins, anti-early embryonic antigens, and anti-human chorionic gonadotropin (hCG).

• This paper discusses advantages and disadvantages of various methods to developing immuno-contraceptive vaccines.

396.

Contraception vaccine stimulates antibody to chorionic gonadotropin. *JAMA* 1977 Feb 7; 237(6): 519-20. [No authors listed.]

"A contraception vaccine which stimulates antibody to chorionic gonadotropin is showing promise in preliminary studies carried out...at the All-India Institute of Medical Sciences."

• The Population Council at Rockefeller University in New York described several obstacles the Indian researchers had to overcome.

• Some tests with rhesus monkeys suggested that the vaccine can prevent pregnancy. However, preliminary experiments on women did not determine whether the antibody will neutralize the biologic function of the hormone.

397.

The World Health Organization has been developing immunologically-based birth control vaccines since 1972

"This account of the activities of the Task Force on Vaccines for Fertility Regulation summarizes the research supported by the World Health Organization...and reflects the long-term, high risk nature of this line of new product development which combines two of the most difficult and sensitive areas of biomedical research, namely, the development of novel vaccines and new methods of birth control."

Griffin PD. **The WHO Task Force on Vaccines for Fertility Regulation. Its formation, objectives and research activities.** *Hum Reprod* 1991 Jan; 6(1): 166-72.

- In 1972, the World Health Organization established the *Special Programme of Research, Development and Research Training in Human Reproduction* to support the development of new contraceptive methods.

- WHO's Special Programme formed several Task Forces, each consisting of an international group of scientists collaborating on predetermined goals.

- In its first year of operation, WHO established the *Task Force on Methods for the Regulation of Implantation* to conduct studies on ways to immunologically prevent an embryo from adhering to the uterus.

- Shortly thereafter, WHO established the *Task Force on Immunological Methods for the Regulation of Fertility* to determine ways to immunologically prevent implantation, inhibit sperm transport and fertilization, and hinder blastocyst hatching through interference with the zona pellucida.

- In 1974, scientists at a WHO-sponsored symposium (in Stockholm) agreed that by neutralizing some reproductive-specific molecules, endocrine or other metabolic disturbances could possibly lead to long-term immunopathology.

- In addition to WHO, major contributors in the field include the Population Council (established by John Rockefeller III in 1952), the National Institutes of Health (USA), and the National Institute of Immunology (India).

398.

When anti-fertility vaccines become more widely available, nations may be tempted to institute population control programs

"As governments grapple with the economic, social, and ecological consequences of population growth, draconian measures to control fertility will be ever more tempting."

Schrater AF. **Immunization to regulate fertility: biological and cultural frameworks.** *Soc Sci Med* 1995 Sep; 41(5): 657-71.

- In 1972, the World Health Organization established a Special Programme to research and develop vaccines to regulate fertility, with an emphasis on the needs of developing countries. The Population Council in New York City was instrumental in helping to formulate contraceptive vaccines.

- This paper analyzed biological, cultural, and gender-related factors that influence beliefs and attitudes associated with anti-fertility vaccines.

- Fertility-regulating vaccines could offer women freedom of choice to prevent their own pregnancies or may be abused by the state to coercively decrease the fertility rate of a population.

- Traditional vaccines target "non-self" antigens. In contrast, some contraceptive vaccines target "self" hormones, which could induce autoimmune disease.

- From a scientist's perspective, vaccines that control birth are similar to those that control disease: both prevent a particular condition.

- Scientists who develop contraceptive vaccines emphasize their advantages while women who might use them cite disadvantages: lack of user control, no signal when protection has begun, inability to turn off an immune response, side-effects, and the potential for misuse by population control programs.

- Population control programs are driven by issues of national welfare, with the well-being of the individual overridden by demands of the state.

- Pregnancy should not be treated like a disease that is subject to state control.

399.

There is opposition to further research on population control vaccines

"Population control ideology should not guide the development of contraceptives. The aim must be to enable women to exert greater control over their fertility without sacrificing their integrity, health, and well being."

Richter J. **Anti-fertility 'vaccines': a plea for an open debate on the prospects of research.** *Newsl Womens Glob Netw Reprod Rights* 1994 Apr-Jun; (46): 3-5.

- The director of the World Health Organization's *Human Reproduction Programme* believes that resistance to anti-fertility vaccine research is largely due to scientific distortions and alarmist speculation.

- The author of this paper argues that safe, reversible immunological contraception is improbable. Once developed, anti-fertility vaccines will be misused and their potential for abuse is sufficient reason to end further research.

400.

Kumar S. **Research into anti-fertility vaccine continues despite protests.** *Lancet* 1998 Nov 7; 352(9139): 1528.

" 'The efficacy profile of these vaccines cannot justify exposing women to potential adverse effects' such as autoimmune diseases...or permanent infertility."

- Protesters at the *International Congress of Reproductive Immunology* (in New Delhi, India) demanded a complete end to all research on anti-fertility vaccines. They claimed that immuno-contraceptives have low efficacy and immune responses cannot be switched off if an adverse reaction occurs.

- Phase I and II trials have already been conducted. To prevent pregnancy, three injections at monthly intervals are required, followed by boosters and monthly antibody titer checks. Judith Richter, with the *International Campaign Against Population Control,* claimed that informed consent norms were disregarded.

401.

Women of reproductive age in several developing nations might have received multiple doses of an anti-fertility vaccine without their consent

"If indeed the purpose of the mass vaccinations is to prevent pregnancies, women are uninformed, unsuspecting, and unconsenting victims."

Tetanus vaccine may be laced with anti-fertility drug. International / developing countries. *Vaccine Wkly* 1995 May 29-Jun 5: 9-10. [No authors listed.]

- The president of Human Life International (HLI) has asked Congress to investigate reports of women in some developing countries unknowingly receiving a tetanus vaccine laced with an anti-fertility drug.

- In 1994, the Pro-Life Committee of Mexico became suspicious of the protocols for a tetanus vaccine campaign because they excluded all males and called for *multiple* injections of the vaccine in women of reproductive age even though *one* injection is protective for at least ten years.

- The Committee had vials of the tetanus vaccine analyzed for human chorionic gonadotropin (hCG), a natural hormone needed to maintain pregnancy. A vaccine laced with hCG would produce antibodies preventing pregnancy.

- Tetanus vaccines laced with hCG also were discovered in the Philippines and Nicaragua.

- Organizations involved in the development of an anti-fertility vaccine using hCG include the World Health Organization (WHO), the United Nations Population Fund, the World Bank, the Rockefeller Foundation, and the United States National Institute of Child Health and Human Development.

402.

The World Health Organization developed a birth control vaccine that might have been tested on unsuspecting pregnant women

"Laboratory testing of the tetanus toxoid vaccine used in the WHO Kenya campaign 2013-2015 showed that some of the vials contained a tetanus toxoid/βhCG conjugate consistent with the WHO's goal to develop one or more anti-fertility vaccines to reduce the rate of population growth, especially in targeted less developed countries such as Kenya."

Oller JW, Shaw CA, et al. **HCG found in WHO tetanus vaccine in Kenya raises concern in the developing world.** *Open Access Library Journal* 2017 Oct; 4(10): 1-32.

- This paper provides evidence that the World Health Organization (WHO) developed an anti-fertility "tetanus" vaccine which was then administered to unsuspecting pregnant girls and women in Kenya.

- Published research since 1972 shows that WHO scientists were able to combine tetanus toxoid with human chorionic gonadotropin (hCG) causing the immune system to attack pregnancy hormones. Expected results are miscarriages and infertility.

- From 2013-2015, pregnant females in Kenya received multiple doses of a vaccine that they believed would protect their babies against neonatal tetanus. However, WHO utilized a dosage schedule appropriate for their anti-fertility birth-control vaccine but inappropriate for a tetanus toxoid vaccine.

- Two Kenyan physicians who participated in the WHO vaccination campaign took vials of the vaccine to multiple WHO-certified laboratories for analyses. More than half were found to contain hCG. (Samples later provided by WHO to the "Joint Committee of Experts" tested negative for hCG.)

- Pro-life organizations have published suspicions since the early 1990s that WHO was vaccinating pregnant women in third world nations with an anti-fertility vaccine under the guise of eliminating neonatal tetanus.

403.

Several birth control vaccines are under development for effective management of the human population

"For effective management of the human population, scientists have been working on the feasibility of developing contraceptive vaccines."

Gupta SK, Shrestha A, Minhas V. **Milestones in contraceptive vaccines development and hurdles in their application.** *Hum Vaccin Immunother* 2014; 10(4): 911-25.

- The increasing human population, especially in developing nations of Asia and Africa, depletes natural resources, jeopardizing food security, drinking water, and the environment.

- This paper reviews significant achievements and hurdles associated with the development of contraceptive vaccines for managing and controlling both human and wildlife populations.

- Contraceptive vaccines are designed to work by inducing a humoral and/or cell-mediated immune response against hormones/proteins that are crucial to reproduction. Ideally, the elicited immune response will nullify their normal biological activity thus preventing fertility.

- Contraceptive vaccines can be categorized into three groups, those that either block the production of sperm and eggs, induce an immune response against sperm- or egg-specific proteins, or neutralize human chorionic gonadotropin (hCG), which is critical to sustaining conception.

- Scientists have several challenges to overcome. For example, the immune response against pregnancy should last at least one year and be reversible. Also, immune responses among vaccinated subjects are variable, so women will need to have their antibody titers monitored to plan for booster shots.

- Contraceptive vaccines that generate antibodies against 'self' proteins must be proven safe with long-term studies. Also, if the vaccine fails and a child is born, potential adverse effects on the child's health will need to be assessed over many years before the vaccine can be recommended for human use.

404.

Anti-fertility vaccine efficacy correlates with the likelihood of developing ovarian dysfunction

"Ovarian suppression may be an inherent feature of effective zona pellucida-based immunocontraception, associated with the generation of elevated antibody titres over a prolonged period of time."

Joonè CJ, Schulman ML, Bertschinger HJ. **Ovarian dysfunction associated with zona pellucida-based immunocontraceptive vaccines.** *Theriogenology* 2017 Feb; 89: 329-37.

• Scientists have been developing an anti-fertility vaccine that targets the zona pellucida (essential for oocyte growth and fertilization). However, this vaccine causes ovarian dysfunction in several animals species. This paper speculates on what is causing the ovarian dysfunction.

• Animal studies showed a direct correlation between the efficacy of the vaccine and ovarian pathology. Conversely, when the vaccine has a poor anti-fertility effect, there is little evidence of ovarian dysfunction.

405.

Hasegawa A, Tanaka H, Shibahara H. **Infertility and immunocontraception based on zona pellucida.** *Reprod Med Biol* 2013 Jun; 13(1): 1-9.

"Immunocontraceptive vaccine development for human use is a long way from achieving satisfactory efficacy and safety."

• The zona pellucida (ZP) is an extracellular membrane that surrounds ovarian eggs and pre-implantation embryos. It is essential to mammalian reproduction. This paper describes the history of immunocontraceptive vaccines involving the ZP and summarizes studies that have utilized this technology.

• Vaccines that utilize ZP antigens elevate anti-ZP antibody levels, which in turn increase the risk of ovarian autoimmune disease and infertility.

406.

Scientists are concerned that birth control vaccines may cause permanent infertility, autoimmune disease, and birth defects

"The theoretical risks involved in the use of anti-fertility vaccines are of two general types. One is the possibility of teratogenic effects.... The other is the possibility of acute and chronic effects in the user. These fall into two categories: endocrinological effects, including possible changes in ovarian and pituitary function, and immunological effects."

Mauck CP, Thau RB. **Safety of anti-fertility vaccines.** *Curr Opin Immunol* 1989; 2(5): 728-32.

- In this paper, scientists associated with the Population Council at New York's Rockefeller University reviewed studies on the potential risks associated with anti-fertility vaccines.

- Safety concerns under discussion were those associated with anti-fertility vaccines using antigens derived from sperm, zona pellucida, human chorionic gonadotropin (hCG), and luteinizing hormone-releasing hormone.

- Scientists are concerned that an immune response to the reproductive antigen could persist, resulting in permanent infertility.

- Immuno-contraceptive vaccines might also induce unexpected cross-reactions between circulating antibodies and non-targeted components of the body, which could result in an autoimmune disease.

- If anti-fertility vaccines fail or the mother discontinues using them and decides to become pregnant, scientists worry about the possibility of teratogenic effects, which could lead to fetal harm and birth defects.

- A comprehensive discussion of anti-fertility vaccine safety issues will be included in a published report of the World Health Organization's *Symposium on Assessing the Safety and Efficacy of Vaccines to Regulate Fertility* held in Geneva, Switzerland, 1989.

407.

There are valid concerns about the safety and ethics of giving women immune-stimulating birth control vaccines

"Women's groups and health activists globally oppose the 'vaccine-approach' to contraception that treats pregnancy as a disease."

Saheli Women's Health Centre. **Research on anti-fertility vaccines: serious concerns for women's health.** *Issues Med Ethics* 2000 Apr-Jun; 8(2): 51-2.

- There is considerable controversy surrounding scientific research to develop immune-stimulating vaccines that control women's fertility.

- This paper highlights unethical and unsound research on immune-stimulating anti-fertility vaccines. It also reveals health risks that immuno-contraceptives pose for women, and the social implications of their use.

- Traditional vaccines target *foreign* antigens. In contrast, anti-fertility vaccines attack *self* antigens that are essential to reproduction. Thus, they have the potential to induce an autoimmune disease.

- Anti-fertility vaccines must be reversible to re-allow conception but the long-term effects of switching the immune status of the body on and off has not been scientifically evaluated.

- Despite decades of anti-fertility vaccine research, failure rates are too high, immune safety and long-term toxicity have not been established, fetal risks are unclear, and there is concern about a potential for permanent infertility.

- Anti-fertility vaccines involve both the immune system and the reproductive system so it is imperative that women be systematically followed up for a sufficient length of time to assess side-effects.

- Many of the anti-fertility vaccine clinical trials have disregarded ethical norms and shown little regard for women's health.

- Women already have numerous safe and effective contraceptive options.

Contaminated Vaccines

The studies in this chapter show that vaccines are sometimes contaminated with unintended potentially dangerous substances. Whether its inorganic elements such as lead, tin, and arsenic, or glyphosate (the active ingredient in herbicides), no one wants foreign matter in human vaccines. DNA fragments of infectious pig viruses were discovered in rotavirus vaccines (which are made using the pancreas of pigs). The monkey virus, SV-40, contaminated polio vaccines that were given to more than 100 million people worldwide. SV-40 causes mesotheliomas, lymphomas, brain tumors, and bone cancer.

408.

Vaccines are contaminated with non-biodegradable particles of barium, copper, iron, lead, tin, and other inorganic elements

"The inorganic particles identified are neither biocompatible nor biodegradable...they are biopersistent.... As happens with all foreign bodies, particularly that small, they induce an inflammatory reaction that is chronic because most of those particles cannot be degraded."

Gatti AM, Montanari S. **New quality-control investigations on vaccines: micro- and nanocontamination.** *Int J Vaccines Vaccin* 2017 Jan 23; 4(1): 7-14.

- In this study, scientists used an environmental scanning electron microscope (equipped with an energy dispersive x-ray spectroscope) to examine 44 vaccine samples to determine whether they were contaminated with foreign matter.

- Several inorganic contaminants (from 100 nanometers to about 10 microns) were identified in human vaccines, including aluminum, antimony, barium, bismuth, bromine, calcium, cerium, chlorine, chromium, copper, gold, hafnium, iron, lead, magnesium, nickel, phosphorous, platinum, potassium, silicon, silver, strontium, sulphur, tin, titanium, tungsten, vanadium, zinc, and zirconium.

- All samples of human vaccines contained lead or stainless steel (iron, chromium and nickel). Only one sample, a veterinarian vaccine, was not contaminated.

- Gardasil samples contained aluminum, barium, bismuth, chlorine, copper, iron, lead, silicon, sulphur, titanium, and zirconium. MMR samples were contaminated with aluminum, barium, bismuth, chromium, copper, iron, lead, nickel, platinum, silicon, silver, sulphur, titanium, tungsten, and vanadium.

- Nano- and micro-sized particles found in vaccines are toxic, induce an inflammatory reaction, and can enter cell nuclei to interact with DNA.

- Multiple contaminants may cause an unpredictable synergistic toxicity.

- Vaccine product inserts did not list the presence of nano- and micro-sized, inorganic foreign matter.

409.

Vaccines are contaminated with glyphosate, the active ingredient in herbicides

"Most disturbing is the presence of glyphosate in many popular vaccines including the measles, mumps and rubella (MMR) vaccine, which we have verified here for the first time. Contamination may come through bovine protein, bovine calf serum, bovine casein, egg protein and/or gelatin. Gelatin sourced from the skin and bones of pigs and cattle given glyphosate-contaminated feed contains the herbicide."

Samsel A, Seneff S. **Glyphosate pathways to modern diseases VI: prions, amyloidoses and autoimmune neurological diseases.** *Journal of Biological Physics and Chemistry* 2017 Mar 15; 17(1): 8-32.

- Glyphosate is the active ingredient in Roundup and other herbicides used on agricultural produce, public land, and residential yards to control weeds.

- This paper explains how glyphosate could replace glycine during protein synthesis, causing a malfunction in the breakdown of proteins into amino acids that could lead to autoimmune disease through molecular mimicry.

- Since pigs and cattle may be fed glyphosate-contaminated forages sprayed with Roundup, contamination may come through live-virus vaccines that are made with bovine calf serum, bovine casein, and gelatin (a common stabilizer in vaccines derived from the skin and bones of pigs and cattle).

- Nineteen different vaccines from five manufacturers were analyzed for glyphosate. All of the vaccines that listed gelatin as an excipient tested positive, including vaccines for chickenpox, shingles, and MMR.

- The MMR vaccine, which contains hydrolyzed gelatin plus fetal bovine serum albumin, human serum albumin, and residual chick embryo, contained the highest levels of glyphosate, significantly more than other vaccines.

- Severe adverse reactions to MMR have increased significantly concurrent with the increased use of glyphosate, a pervasive herbicide which may be associated with digestive enzyme inhibition, gluten intolerance, multiple sclerosis, inflammatory bowel disease, type 1 diabetes, and autism.

410.

Aluminum adjuvants in vaccines contain elemental impurities that cause antigen degradation and loss of vaccine potency

"Trace amounts of residual metal impurities were observed in commercially available aluminum hydroxide lots obtained from various suppliers."

Schlegl R, Weber M, et al. **Influence of elemental impurities in aluminum hydroxide adjuvant on the stability of inactivated Japanese Encephalitis vaccine, IXIARO®**. *Vaccine* 2015 Nov 4; 33(44): 5989-96.

- In this paper, scientists analyzed samples of aluminum hydroxide (a common adjuvant used in vaccines) to identify trace quantities of elemental impurities and determine whether they affect antigen stability.

- Several elemental impurities were identified in aluminum hydroxide samples, including arsenic, barium, chromium, cobalt, copper, iron, gallium, lanthanum, lead, molybdenum, nickel, strontium, tungsten, vanadium, and zirconium.

- There were significant differences in types and quantities of elemental impurities found in aluminum hydroxide, varying between commercial suppliers, but also between different lots from the same supplier.

- Differences in the content and quantity of residual metal impurities could be due to variations in raw materials used, such as the sources of aluminum salts, and proprietary production processes of individual manufacturers.

- A large loss of vaccine potency due to antigen instability and degradation can occur from elemental impurities in aluminum hydroxide adjuvant.

- Antigen degradation was demonstrated to occur via auto-oxidation of sulfite, through the formation of reactive free radicals, catalyzed by the residual metal impurity copper — even at low parts per million (ppm).

- This study showed that vaccines are contaminated with trace metals which are capable of inciting degradation of the vaccine antigen, which must remain potent to stimulate immunity against a particular pathogen and disease.

411.

Adventitious agents, including monkey and pig viruses, contaminated vaccines

"In all four cases...the vaccines concerned were not removed from the market, or were only temporarily suspended, since the benefits of immunization were believed to be much more beneficial than the risk of any potential adverse effects."

Petricciani J, Sheets R, et al. **Adventitious agents in viral vaccines: lessons learned from 4 case studies.** *Biologicals* 2014 Sep; 42(5): 223-36.

- Vaccines are sometimes accidentally contaminated with potentially dangerous adventitious agents. In this paper, researchers analyzed regulatory actions associated with four instances where licensed viral vaccines were found to contain a contaminating agent.

- The four cases analyzed in this paper include: 1) SV40 (simian virus #40) found in polio vaccines, 2) bacteriophages in measles vaccines, 3) reverse transcriptase in measles and mumps vaccines, and 4) porcine circovirus and porcine circovirus DNA sequences in rotavirus vaccines.

- By 1961, it was known that monkey kidneys used to make polio vaccines were contaminated with SV40, a cancer-causing monkey virus. Studies confirmed that SV40 was infectious to humans yet the National Institutes of Health (NIH) recommended that polio vaccine programs continue unabated.

- In 1973, live bacterial viruses (bacteriophages) that could potentially induce multiple human diseases were found in measles vaccines. The FDA responded by permitting the phages in the vaccines, reassuring the public of vaccine safety, and recommending that measles vaccine programs continue unabated.

- In 1995, an avian retrovirus "with unknown safety implications" was found in the MMR vaccine. No regulatory action was taken by either the FDA or WHO to prevent the use of chicken-cell-derived vaccines, still in use today.

- In 2010, DNA fragments of infectious pig viruses were discovered in rotavirus vaccines (which are made using the pancreas of pigs). Vaccine use was not halted because "any risk was outweighed by the benefit of the vaccines."

412.

Polio vaccines were contaminated with monkey viruses that cause brain tumors and possibly AIDS

"Is it only a coincidence that HIV infection manifested itself at the same time as the introduction of vaccines that are now known to have been contaminated with simian viruses?"

Elswood BF, Stricker RB. **Polio vaccines and the origin of AIDS.** *Medical Hypothesis* 1994 Jun; 42(6): 347-354.

- In 1960, researchers discovered that both the inactivated and live polio vaccines had been contaminated with a monkey virus, SV-40. Up to 30 million US citizens and hundreds of millions of people worldwide were affected.

- SV-40 was shown to cause brain tumors at a rate 13 times greater among children of mothers who had received the tainted polio vaccine.

- The AIDS pandemic may have originated from a polio vaccine tainted with SIV, a monkey virus that is similar to HIV, administered to Africans.

413.

Carbone M, Gazdar A, Butel JS. **SV40 and human mesothelioma.** *Trans Lung Cancer Res* 2020; 9(Suppl 1): S47-S59.

"Numerous studies verified the presence of SV40 DNA sequences in brain tumors, mesotheliomas, lymphomas, and osteosarcomas."

- Polio vaccines were grown in rhesus monkey kidney cells that contained SV40. They contaminated many lots of polio vaccines between 1955-1963.

- SV40 has been linked to brain cancers, bone cancers, and lymphomas.

- Analysis of 15 studies shows that SV40 affects cancer patients 15 times more than controls (OR = 15.1). It increases the risk or brain cancer, non-Hodgkin lymphoma, and bone cancer, with ORs of 3.8, 5.4, and 24.5, respectively.

Additional Studies

The studies in this chapter cover a variety of topics. Most people don't realize that vaccines increase the risk of neuropsychiatric disorders, including obsessive-compulsive disorder, attention-deficit hyperactivity disorder, anorexia, anxiety, and tic disorder. Vaccines also contain food proteins that cause food allergies. Lyons-Weiler found that doctors who allow families to accept or reject vaccines sacrifice profits and risk losing their license to practice medicine. Elisha found that studies critical of vaccines may get retracted to stifle dissent and protect the monetary interests of the vaccine industry. These are just some of the topics covered in this section.

414.

Vaccines increase the risk of neuro-psychiatric disorders, including OCD, ADHD, anorexia, anxiety and tic disorder

"This pilot epidemiologic analysis implies that the onset of some neuropsychiatric disorders may be temporally related to prior vaccinations in a subset of individuals."

Leslie DL, Kobre RA, et al. **Temporal association of certain neuro-psychiatric disorders following vaccination of children and adolescents: a pilot case-control study.** *Front Psychiatry* 2017 Jan 19; 8: 3.

- In this paper, children 6-15 years of age with a diagnosis of obsessive-compulsive disorder (OCD), attention deficit hyperactivity disorder (ADHD), anorexia nervosa, anxiety disorder, tic disorder, major depression, or bipolar disorder were compared to age and gender matched controls.

- Subjects who were recently diagnosed with anorexia nervosa were significantly more likely than controls to have received any vaccination within the previous 3-month period (hazard ratio, HR = 1.80).

- Subjects who were recently diagnosed with OCD, ADHD, anorexia nervosa, anxiety disorder, or tic disorder were significantly more likely than controls to have received any vaccination within the previous 6- and 12-month periods.

- Children with OCD, anorexia nervosa, anxiety disorder, or tic disorder were significantly more likely to have received an influenza vaccine during the previous 1-year period.

- Hepatitis A, meningitis, and tetanus-diphtheria vaccines were also associated with significant increases in the risk of neuropsychiatric disorders.

- A higher percentage of females were diagnosed with anorexia (86.6%) and major depression (56.3%). More males were diagnosed with tic disorder (76.4%), ADHD (66.8%), OCD (56.6%), and bipolar disorder (54.1%).

- This study was approved by the Penn State College of Medicine Institutional Review Board.

415.

Vaccines contain food proteins that cause food allergies

"Applying prudent avoidance means we should immediately stop multiple vaccines being administered simultaneously. It is likely to reduce the probability of developing food allergies by reducing the amount of food proteins and adjuvants that are injected at one time."

Arumugham V. **Evidence that food proteins in vaccines cause the development of food allergies and its implications for vaccine policy.** *J Develop Drugs* 2015 Oct 10; 4(4): 137.

- Many vaccines contain food proteins. When a protein is injected into animals or humans, the immune system is sensitized to that protein. Subsequent exposure to the protein can cause anaphylaxis or allergic reactions.

- The National Academy of Medicine (formerly the Institute of Medicine) confirmed that food proteins in vaccines cause food allergies.

- Food proteins found in vaccines include chicken egg (ovalbumin), casamino acids (or casein), gelatin, soy, and agar. Ovalbumin can sensitize to egg. Casamino acid is derived from milk proteins and induces allergy to dairy.

- Vaccines also contain polysorbate 80 and sorbitol which are manufactured from food sources. For example, polysorbate 80 may come from coconut, palm, sunflower, tapioca, wheat, or corn oil.

- Vaccines also contain adjuvants such as pertussis toxins and aluminum that can increase the immunogenicity of injected food proteins.

- Children receive several vaccines concurrently with numerous food proteins and adjuvants injected at one time, increasing the risk of allergic sensitization.

- Allergens in vaccines are not adequately disclosed and no safe dosages or regulations have been established.

- There is a food allergy epidemic. Food allergies from vaccines may take months to diagnose. Food proteins in vaccines should be removed.

416.

First-born children have more emergency room visits following vaccination than later-born children

"Birth order is associated with increased incidence of emergency room (ER) visits and hospitalizations following vaccination in infancy. First-born children had significantly higher relative incidence of events compared to later-born children."

Hawken S, Kwong JC, et al. **Association between birth order and emergency room visits and acute hospital admissions following pediatric vaccination: a self-controlled study.** *PloS One* 2013 Dec 4; 8(12): e81070.

- This study was designed to determine whether adverse events following recommended vaccines, as measured by ER visits and hospitalizations, is associated with the vaccinated child's birth order in the family.

- Birth and health data on more than 274,000 infants was compiled. Adverse events within a pre-specified risk period were compared to a control period following vaccination. The relative incidence of adverse events for first-born versus later-born children was calculated.

- First-born children were significantly more likely than later born children to have ER visits or hospital admissions following their vaccines.

- For the 2-month vaccines, first-born children had a 37% increase in ER visits or hospital admissions compared to later-born children. For the 4-month vaccines, first-born children had a 70% increase in ER visits or hospital admissions compared to later-born children.

- For the 12-month vaccines, there were 249 additional ER visits or hospital admissions for every 100,000 vaccinated first-borns compared to later-borns.

- Excess post-vaccination ER visits may be due to heightened parental concern typical of first-time parents, physiological differences, unknown maternal factors, or the "hygiene hypothesis" which postulates that later-born children with more siblings and exposure to infections may gain immune benefits.

417.

Adverse events following vaccination are affected by the month in which the vaccinated child is born

"We investigated the impact of month of birth on the relative incidence of adverse events following immunization using emergency room visits and hospital admissions as a proxy. Our study is, to the best of our knowledge, the first to describe a seasonal effect of susceptibility to adverse events following immunization."

Hawken S, Potter BK, et al. **Seasonal variation in rates of emergency room visits and acute admissions following recommended infant vaccinations in Ontario, Canada: a self-controlled case series analysis.** *Vaccine* 2014 Dec 12; 32(52): 7148-53.

- This study was designed to determine whether a child's birth month has an effect on the incidence of adverse events following recommended vaccines.

- Birth and health data on more than one million newborns was compiled. The relative incidence of emergency room visits and hospitalizations within a pre-specified risk period were then compared to a control period following vaccination.

- Infants born in April were twice as likely as those born in October to visit an emergency room or be admitted to a hospital after receiving their 2-month vaccinations (relative incidence ratio, RIR = 2.06).

- Infants born in July were significantly more likely than those born in November to visit an emergency room or be admitted to a hospital after receiving their 12-month MMR vaccination (RIR = 1.52).

- The findings in this study may be attributable to birth month, vaccination month, or a combination of the two.

- The authors speculate that variations in sunlight exposure (and circulating vitamin D levels) by season during sensitive periods of fetal and perinatal growth could influence immune development in early life, causing variations in the risk of immune-related problems and adverse vaccine reactions.

316 of Miller's Review of Critical Vaccine Studies, Volume 2

418.

The World Health Organization gave children a dangerous malaria vaccine without parental knowledge or consent

"Parents should be made aware of this doubled female mortality....
Recipients of the malaria vaccine are not being informed that they are
in a study.... No person shall be subjected to medical or scientific
experimentation without his or her consent."

Doshi P. **WHO's malaria vaccine study represents a "serious breach of international ethical standards."** *BMJ* 2020 Feb 26; 368: m734.

- In a Phase III clinical trial of a new malaria vaccine, Mosquirix, vaccinated children had a 10-fold increase in meningitis and a 2-fold increase in cerebral malaria, compared to unvaccinated children. All-cause mortality in vaccinated girls was twice as high as in the control group (relative risk, RR = 2.00).

- Despite these safety concerns, the World Health Organization (WHO) implemented a clandestine study and mass vaccination program in Malawi, Ghana, and Kenya where 720,000 children were expected to receive this new malaria vaccine.

- The parents of these children were unaware that they were taking part in this study which was designed to further assess the safety of this new vaccine. The parents were not informed of the safety concerns discovered in the Phase III clinical trial. The parents were unable to give their informed consent.

- WHO claimed that the physical presence of the child during vaccination, with or without an accompanying parent, "is considered to imply consent."

- Previous studies of five other non-live vaccines have already shown an association with increased female mortality.

- The failure of WHO to require informed consent prior to enrolling children in a randomized study with a vaccine that has already provided evidence of increased mortality and other safety concerns is a serious breach of international ethical standards.

419.

Health professionals who administer vaccines to adults must first obtain informed consent free of duress

"An adult person of sound mind is entitled to decide which, if any, of the available forms of immunization to undergo, and their consent has to be obtained before immunization is undertaken. There is now a duty to take reasonable care to ensure that a patient is aware of any material risks involved in any recommended immunization, and of any reasonable alternative or variant to immunization. Health professionals can no longer selectively choose what information to disclose."

Griffith R. **Obtaining consent for the immunization of adults.** *Hum Vaccin Immunother* 2016; 12(1): 231-34.

- This paper discusses legal obligations of health professionals who administer vaccines to adults.

- Since 1914, the right to self-determination and principles of informed consent were established in law. Schloendorff v. Society of New York Hospital held that "every human being of adult years and sound mind has a right to determine what shall be done with their own body."

- Health professionals are required by law to explain the risks of vaccination, a duty founded in the law of negligence. The adult patient is also entitled to information about alternative treatments.

- Health professionals cannot force or deceive an unwilling competent adult into having a vaccine because that would be a crime.

- To protect health professionals from liability and preserve the legal rights of the adult, consent must be obtained prior to vaccination.

- Consent may be written or verbal. To be valid, consent must be free from duress and reasonably informed.

- Consent must be freely chosen by the individual. Excessive influence from family or health professionals invalidates the consent.

420.

Adverse events following vaccination are more common in children of lower socioeconomic status

"Our study identified that lower socioeconomic status increased the likelihood of an adverse event following vaccination."

Wilson K, Ducharme R, Hawken S. **Association between socioeconomic status and adverse events following immunization at 2, 4, 6 and 12 months.** *Hum Vaccin Immunother* 2013 May; 9(5): 1153-57.

- This study was designed to determine whether adverse events following recommended vaccines, as measured by emergency room visits and hospital admissions, is associated with the vaccinated child's socioeconomic status.

- Health and socioeconomic data on more than 1.2 million infants was compiled. Adverse events within a pre-specified risk period were compared to a control period following vaccination. The relative incidence of adverse events for children of lower versus higher socioeconomic status was calculated.

- Children living in families with the lowest incomes were significantly more likely than children living in families with the highest incomes to have adverse events following their 12-month MMR vaccination ($p = .02$).

- Lower socioeconomic status was also associated with a significantly increased risk of adverse events following their 4-month vaccinations ($p = .03$).

- The top diagnoses for emergency room visits and hospital admissions were acute respiratory infection, otitis media, non-infective colitis/gastroenteritis, unspecified viral infection, and unspecified fever.

- The authors speculate that real physiological differences might exist between children of lower and higher socioeconomic status. Low income is a known risk factor for nutritional deficiencies which could affect immune responses and increase adverse events following vaccination.

421.

Pertussis vaccines for adolescents fail to protect against epidemics of the disease

"This study demonstrates that despite high rates of Tdap vaccination, the growing cohort of adolescents who have only received acellular pertussis vaccines continue to be at high risk of contracting pertussis and sustaining epidemics."

Klein NP, Bartlett J, et al. **Waning Tdap effectiveness in adolescents.** *Pediatrics* 2016 Mar; 137(3): e20153326.

- In the USA, children receive 5 doses of an acellular pertussis vaccine (DTaP). They receive another acellular pertussis vaccine (Tdap) during adolescence.

- In this study, scientists examined Tdap vaccine effectiveness among adolescents previously vaccinated exclusively with DTaP. (They did not receive any doses of DTP, the whole-cell pertussis vaccine.)

- Tdap did not prevent pertussis outbreaks. Although 96.5% of teens in California had received Tdap by age 14, there were epidemics of pertussis.

- Tdap vaccine efficacy was 69% during the first year after vaccination, declining to 57% during the second year, 25% in the third year, and 9% in the fourth year and beyond.

- During recent pertussis outbreaks, the risk of pertussis in teens who received Tdap increased by an average of 35% per year following vaccination.

- There was no significant difference in the incidence rate of pertussis between Tdap-vaccinated and Tdap-unvaccinated populations (ages 10-19 years).

- Because pertussis transmission is affected by variations in both vaccine efficacy and pertussis transmission rates, control of whooping cough is not possible by simply providing high vaccine coverage in the right age groups.

- Because Tdap does not generate long-term protection against pertussis, it may be more effective to provide the shot prior to the expectation of a local pertussis outbreak instead of on a routine basis.

422.

Vaccine mandates are not recommended

"Current attitudes of public health officials about vaccine mandates and exemptions are arrogant and patronizing."

Cunningham AS. **Vaccine mandates in the US are doing more harm than good.** *BMJ* 2015 Aug; 351: h4576. [Commentary.]

- Following an outbreak of measles in the U.S., a lot of media became malicious toward parents who obtain non-medical exemptions. Health officials have lost perspective regarding families that obtain vaccine exemptions.

- Professional and financial incentives encourage strict adherence to the vaccine schedule. Health authorities tend to report positive findings about vaccines but ignore bad news.

- Many vaccine studies are sponsored by the manufacturers and are designed mainly to demonstrate short-term efficacy with little effort toward finding serious adverse reactions.

- Public health colleagues in Canada perceive serious ethical problems in the vaccine approval process. Vaccine manufacturers and professionals with close ties to industry should not be involved in lobbying and decision making.

- The concept of herd immunity has been used to bully parents into rigid adherence to the recommended vaccine schedule.

- Mathematical models estimate that from 55% to 96% of children need to be vaccinated to prevent the spread of measles. Yet, officials use these *measles* simulations to foster public disapproval of parents who decline *any* vaccine, and to impose mandates.

- Public health officials in the United States want to shrink the number of non-medical exemptions by making it costly and inconvenient for families to obtain them. This is unwise because it will foster mistrust and resistance.

- Knowledge about vaccines is incomplete; some flexibility must be permitted for non-medical vaccine exemptions. Public health officials should not force families into rigid mandates for every vaccine on the schedule.

423.

Doctors who allow families to accept or reject vaccines sacrifice profits and risk losing their license to practice medicine

"Physicians who respect and abide by the principle of informed consent are being persecuted and punished for doing so."

Lyons-Weiler J, Thomas P. **Vaccine practice payment schedules create perverse incentives for unnecessary medical procedures—at what cost to patients?** *Int J of Vaccine Theory, Practice, and Research* 2021 Mar; 2(1): 25-37.

- This paper analyzed the financial and punitive consequences that occur when a medical doctor allows parents to reject vaccines for their children.

- Using data from a pediatric practice that respects informed consent, profits from vaccines administered and losses from vaccines refused were tabulated.

- In a pediatric practice, there are two main sources of profit from vaccines: the markup on the purchase and a fee for administering each vaccine. A busy pediatric practice could gain or lose one million dollars per year on the administration fee alone, depending on whether informed consent is honored.

- Insurance companies incentivize high rates of vaccination through their bonus structures and conditions for reimbursement, leading many pediatricians to discharge patients who reject vaccines. High costs to operate a pediatric practice also act as a financial incentive to increase vaccination rates.

- Physicians who abide by state laws and federal regulations regarding informed consent by allowing parents the option of not vaccinating or not following the CDC vaccine schedule not only sacrifice profits but risk being sanctioned by their medical board and/or losing their license to practice medicine.

- The focus of a pediatric practice should be on the *quality* of health outcomes, not the *quantity* of medical procedures administered. Only doctors who respect a parent's choice are practicing ethical medicine.

424.

Outcome reporting bias in vaccine studies and partisan allegiance to medical consensus hinder public health

"Independent researchers experience an astonishing level of censorship by medical journal editors who deny publication when outcome reporting bias in the original published studies is exposed and re-analysis leads to conclusions contrary to the medical consensus. This conduct obscures medical and scientific truth."

Goldman GS. **Examples of outcome reporting bias in vaccine studies: illustrating how perpetuating medical consensus can impede progress in public health.** *Cureus* 2022 Sep 21; 14(9): e29399.

- Outcome reporting bias—selective reporting of findings that support preset beliefs and desired results—is a widespread problem in vaccine studies. This paper identifies seven vaccine studies with outcome reporting bias and shows how partisan allegiance to medical consensus hinders public health.

- Chief editors of *The Lancet* and *New England Journal of Medicine* have warned that vaccine studies published in peer-reviewed journals contain a high degree of outcome reporting bias and thus appear to serve as a marketing arm of the pharmaceutical industry.

- Outcome reporting bias may occur when data are manipulated until computer programs output selective results that support a preset conclusion. Medical journals may spread false information by preferentially publishing vaccine studies that perpetuate medical consensus despite unreliable findings.

- Conflicts of interest between regulatory agencies and the vaccine industry impact what is deemed to be medical consensus. Their sponsorship of selective studies that often lack data transparency reinforces the dominant narrative.

- Scientists who present factual data and analyses critical of medical consensus are censored for promoting vaccine hesitancy through "misinformation."

- Outcome reporting bias obscures scientific truth. Medical orthodoxy can be wrong. To resolve contradictory findings, research integrity is advocated.

425.

Vaccinated children have significantly more office visits for adverse events than unvaccinated children

"Estimates of health care incidence show that visits above regular health care visits increase due to vaccination by 2.56 to 4.98 additional office visits for vaccine-related health issues per unit increase in vaccination per year."

Lyons-Weiler J, Blaylock RL. **Revisiting excess diagnoses of illnesses and conditions in children whose parents provided informed permission to vaccinate them.** *IJVTPR* 2022 Sep 26; 2(2): 603-18

- Studies finding a link between vaccines and adverse events are often targeted for retraction. One such study, using data from the medical practice of Paul Thomas, MD, was retracted after an anonymous reader alleged that healthcare-seeking behavior varied between vaccinated and unvaccinated populations.

- Office visits between 561 vaccinated and 561 unvaccinated patients were compared. Vaccinated patients had higher rates of office visits ($p < 0.01$) for ear infections (2.94), anemia (OR = 2.57), gastroenteritis (OR = 2.53), eczema (OR = 2.29), and food allergy (OR = 2.00).

- This study revealed that vaccination increases non-routine office visits (not "well-baby visits"), in contrast to the implication that unkept appointments by non-vaccinators led to fewer diagnoses.

- Variation in healthcare-seeking behavior cannot explain the increased need by vaccinated children for non-routine visits to the doctor's office for adverse health conditions.

- Well-designed, peer-reviewed studies should not be retracted based on suppositions unsupported by data.

- Using a variety of methods, this paper shows that the anonymous reader's concerns that led to the retraction was unfounded.

426.

Studies critical of vaccines may get retracted to stifle dissent and protect the monetary interests of the vaccine industry

"These findings point to the need for a fair, open, and honest discourse about the safety of vaccines for the benefit of public health and the restoration of trust in science and medicine."

Elisha E, Guetzkow J, et al. **Retraction of scientific papers: the case of vaccine research.** *Critical Public Health* 2022; 32(4): 533-42.

- Research that contradicts official positions may be suppressed through censorship, restricted access to funding, and by retraction of papers from scientific journals after publication.

- This study examined the perspectives of eight internationally recognized researchers whose scientific papers on vaccine safety problems were retracted.

- Of 24 retracted papers on vaccines, all of them discussed safety concerns. None of the retracted papers had positive findings supporting vaccine safety.

- Anonymous complaints by proxies of the pharmaceutical industry regarding alleged methodological flaws that are minor, irrelevant or false pressure editors of scientific journals to retract papers that challenge pro-vaccine views.

- The researchers in this study perceived the retraction of their papers as a way for the vaccine industry to censor vaccine critics, harm them professionally, label them as anti-vaccinators, and delegitimize their studies as junk science.

- Journalists uncritically perpetuate the pro-vaccine agenda, rarely investigate vaccine safety, but readily denigrate "anti-vaccine" researchers.

- Retractions deter other scientists from participating in research that might reveal vaccine safety concerns, further strengthening the pro-vaccine agenda.

- Retracting valid papers that challenge prevailing ideas is unethical, undermines scientific integrity, narrows our world view, and threatens public health.

Index

About the Author

Neil Z. Miller is a medical research journalist. He has devoted the past 35 years to educating parents and health practitioners about vaccines, encouraging informed consent and non-mandatory laws. He is the author of several books, studies and articles on vaccines, including *Miller's Review of Critical Vaccine Studies* (Volume I), *Vaccine Safety Manual for Concerned Families and Health Practitioners,* and *Vaccines: Are They Really Safe and Effective?* Mr. Miller has a degree in psychology and is a member of Mensa. He lives in New Mexico, USA.

Purchasing Information

Miller's Review of Critical Vaccine Studies, Volume II (ISBN: 978-188121744-2) may be purchased directly from *New Atlantean Press*. Call 505-983-1856. Or send $21.95 (in U.S. funds), plus $5.00 for media mail shipping (or $7.00 for priority shipping) to:

New Atlantean Press
PO Box 9638, Santa Fe, NM 87504
505-983-1856 (Telephone & Fax)
Email: think@thinktwice.com

This book is also available at www.vacbook.com or at many fine bookstores.

Bookstores/Libraries/Retail Buyers: Order from Independent Publisher's Group (IPG), Midpoint, Ingram, Baker &Taylor, or New Atlantean Press.

Parents, Chiropractors, Naturopaths, and other Non-Storefront Buyers: Take a 40% discount with the purchase of 5 or more copies (multiply the total cost of purchases x .60). Please add 9% for shipping. Larger discounts are available. Call or email us for case quantity discounts and shipping rates.

Shipping Rates

United States (1 or 2 books): Please add $5.00 for media mail (allow 1-3 weeks for your order to arrive) or include $2.00 extra ($7.00 total) for Priority shipping.
Canada and Mexico: Please add $24.00 for Global Priority shipping.
Europe, Asia and Australia: Please add $26.00 for Global Priority shipping.

More Vaccine Resources

Miller's Review of Critical Vaccine Studies (Volume I) (ISBN: 978-188121740-4). A premier collection of significant vaccine studies. An indispensable resource. Code: MRO (336 pages) $21.95.

Vaccine Safety Manual for Concerned Families and Health Practitioners, 2nd Edition (ISBN: 978-18812174037-4). The most extensive guide to vaccine-related diseases and vaccine risks. Includes more than 1,000 scientific citations. More than 100 charts, graphs and illustrations supplement the text. This encyclopedic health manual is an important addition to every family's home library and will be referred to again and again. Code: VSM (352 pages) $19.95.

Vaccines: Are They *Really* Safe and Effective? (ISBN: 978-188121730-5). An excellent introductory book on vaccine safety and efficacy issues. Includes 30 charts and more than 900 citations. Code: VAC (128 pages) $12.95.

New Atlantean Press offers additional books and other resources:
www.vacbook.com / www.thinkchoice.com